Practice Questions in Trauma and Orthopaedics for the FRCS

Pankaj Sharma
Specialist Registrar in Trauma and Orthopaedic Surgery
Wessex Rotation, Winchester

Foreword by

Nicola Maffulli
Professor of Trauma and Orthopaedic Surgery
Keele University School of Medicine

Radcliffe Publishing
Oxford ● New York

Radcliffe Publishing Ltd
18 Marcham Road
Abingdon
Oxon OX14 1AA
United Kingdom

www.radcliffe-oxford.com
Electronic catalogue and worldwide online ordering facility.

© 2007 Pankaj Sharma

Pankaj Sharma has asserted his right under the Copyright, Designs and Patents Act 1998 to be identified as the author of this work.

British Library Cataloguing in Publication Data

A catalogue record for this book is available from the British Library.

ISBN-13: 978 1 84619 200 5

Typeset by Advance Typesetting Ltd, Oxford
Printed and bound by TJI Digital, Padstow, Cornwall

Contents

Foreword

Exams never end! This is a sad fact of life, and we can only strive to be well prepared, or better prepared, for the task. Also, practice makes perfect.

Practice Questions in Trauma and Orthopaedics for the FRCS aims to be a comprehensive tool to help in the final assessment for the FRCS (Tr Orth). Mr Sharma is to be congratulated not only for identifying a gap in the orthopaedic literature and the need for a specialist book, but also for successfully producing a comprehensive text to cover the vast subject of trauma and orthopaedics. This is not intended to be exhaustive, and cannot substitute for good old-fashioned reading with teaching and operative and diagnostic skills to match. The questions are up to date, easy to understand and interpret, and follow a logical path. Above all, they seem to reflect the structure of the exam, and can therefore be used as a basis for teaching, as a revision tool, and as a pre-test confidence booster.

Mr Sharma has started something which will keep him occupied for many years. This book will require regular revision to keep it up to date with the rapid growth of orthopaedics and trauma, biochemistry, biomechanics, imaging, and techniques of clinical management.

So, reader, dig in – there is only one way to go, and it is in the depths of this book.

Nicola Maffulli MD, MS, PhD, FRCS (Orth)
Professor of Trauma and Orthopaedic Surgery
Keele University School of Medicine
May 2007

Preface

This book is primarily aimed at Specialist Registrars in Trauma and Orthopaedics, who are preparing for the Fellowship of the Royal College of Surgeons examination. However, it will also be useful for candidates preparing for the MRCS examination. The format of the examination has changed recently, and there will not be any written paper. Instead there will be two papers, consisting of multiple-choice and extended matching questions. I believe that this book will provide valuable revision and practice for candidates taking the FRCS (Tr Orth) examination.

Pankaj Sharma
Specialist Registrar in Trauma and Orthopaedic Surgery
Wessex Rotation, Winchester
May 2007

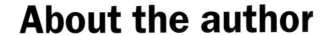

About the author

Pankaj Sharma graduated from the United Medical and Dental Schools of Guy's and St Thomas' Hospitals (UMDS), London in 1997. He did his house jobs in the Kent region, and then undertook a basic surgical training rotation in Cardiff, Wales. During this period he passed his MRCS examination. He subsequently worked as a Junior Clinical Fellow in Trauma and Orthopaedics at King's College Hospital, London. He then undertook a Basic Science Research Fellowship at the University Hospital of North Staffordshire, under the supervision of Professor Nicola Maffulli and Professor Alicia El Haj.

In 2004, he was appointed to the post of Specialist Registrar in Trauma and Orthopaedics on the Wessex Rotation, where he is still currently in post.

He has published extensively in medical journals, and has more than 20 peer-reviewed papers to his credit, along with one book chapter.

Acknowledgements

I am most grateful to Professor Nicola Maffulli for reading through the manuscript of this book, and for his perceptive comments.

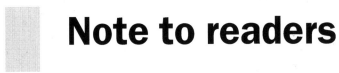

Note to readers

Please note that there is only *one* correct response to each question.

I would like to dedicate this book to my father, for supporting me in every way during my surgical training, and to my wife, Anusha, without whose help and encouragement this book would not have been possible.

Section 1

Basic science

Q1 What percentage of the skeleton does cortical bone account for?

(a) 10%.
(b) 20%.
(c) 40%.
(d) 60%.
(e) 80%.

Q2 Which of the following cell types responds to calcitonin?

(a) Osteocyte.
(b) Osteoclast.
(c) Osteoblast.
(d) Fibroblast.
(e) Osteoprogenitor cell.

Q3 With regard to the physis, which zone has the highest PO_2?

(a) Reserve zone.
(b) Proliferative zone.
(c) Maturation zone.
(d) Zone of provisional calcification.
(e) Degenerative zone.

Q4 Which of the following types of graft has the best osteoconductive properties?

(a) Cancellous autograft.
(b) Cortical autograft.
(c) Bone marrow.

(d) Demineralised bone matrix.

(e) Ceramic.

Q5 Which of the following conditions demonstrates normal bone mineralisation?

(a) Osteomalacia.

(b) Rickets.

(c) Osteoporosis.

(d) Osteopetrosis.

(e) Renal osteodystrophy.

Q6 The active metabolite $1,25\text{-}(OH)_2$ vitamin D is formed after $1\text{-}\alpha$-hydroxylation in which site?

(a) Skin.

(b) Liver.

(c) Small intestine.

(d) Bone.

(e) Kidney.

Q7 What is the predominant type of collagen found in bone?

(a) Type I.

(b) Type II.

(c) Type III.

(d) Type V.

(e) Type XII.

Q8 What is the predominant type of collagen found in articular cartilage?

(a) Type I.

(b) Type II.

(c) Type III.

(d) Type V.

(e) Type XII.

(Q9)   Which of the following zones of articular cartilage is exposed to the highest levels of compressive strain?

(a)   Superficial zone.
(b)   Transitional zone.
(c)   Radial zone.
(d)   Tidemark.
(e)   Calcified zone.

(Q10)   Which of the following is the main mechanism for lubrication of articular joints during dynamic function?

(a)   Weeping lubrication.
(b)   Boosted lubrication.
(c)   Boundary lubrication.
(d)   Elastohydrodynamic lubrication.
(e)   Hydrodynamic lubrication.

(Q11)   Which joint is most commonly affected in osteoarthritis?

(a)   Hip.
(b)   Shoulder.
(c)   Knee.
(d)   Ankle.
(e)   Thumb carpometacarpal joint.

(Q12)   Which of the following changes takes place in articular cartilage in osteoarthritis?

(a)   Increase in collagen content.
(b)   Increase in water content.
(c)   Increase in proteoglycan content.
(d)   Increase in keratin sulphate.
(e)   Increase in modulus of elasticity.

(Q13) During muscle contraction, to which of the following does calcium bind?

(a) Actin.
(b) Myosin.
(c) Tropomycin.
(d) Sarcoplasmic reticulum.
(e) Troponin.

(Q14) Which of the following signs is present in lower motor neuron lesions?

(a) Hypertonia.
(b) Hyperreflexia.
(c) Positive plantar reflex.
(d) Fasciculation.
(e) Clonus.

(Q15) As which of the following is median nerve division at the wrist by a knife classified?

(a) Neurotmesis.
(b) Axonotmesis.
(c) Epineurolysis.
(d) Neuropraxia.
(e) Wallerian degeneration.

(Q16) Due to which of the following does traumatic failure of tendon function most commonly occur?

(a) Osteotendinous junction rupture.
(b) Tendon body rupture.
(c) Musculotendinous junction rupture.
(d) Muscle belly rupture.
(e) Avulsion fracture.

Q17 Which of the following is the first type of immunoglobulin to increase in response to acute infection?

(a) IgA.
(b) IgM.
(c) IgD.
(d) IgE.
(e) IgG.

Q18 In children undergoing surgery for which of the following conditions has latex allergy been reported?

(a) Congenital talipes equinovarus.
(b) Tibial torsion.
(c) Proximal femoral anteversion.
(d) Developmental dysplasia of the hip.
(e) Myelomeningocoele.

Q19 Which of the following agents is the most common causative agent in osteomyelitis?

(a) Group A streptococcus.
(b) *Staphylococcus aureus.*
(c) *Staphylococcus epidermidis.*
(d) *Pseudomonas aeruginosa.*
(e) *Clostridium perfringens.*

Q20 Which of the following is the commonest site at which septic arthritis follows osteomyelitis?

(a) Knee.
(b) Wrist.
(c) Shoulder.
(d) Hip.
(e) Ankle.

Q21 With which of the following should patients with total joint replacements *in situ* who are undergoing dental work have routine antibiotic prophylaxis?

(a) No prophylaxis required.
(b) Co-amoxiclav.
(c) Cephalexin.
(d) Ciprofloxacin.
(e) Teicoplanin.

Q22 Which of the following antibiotics has been associated with a high incidence of pseudomembranous colitis?

(a) Metronidazole.
(b) Chloramphenicol.
(c) Tetracycline.
(d) Imipenem.
(e) Clindamycin.

Q23 Which of the following antibiotics reaches the highest concentration in bone?

(a) Ciprofloxacin.
(b) Teicoplanin.
(c) Vancomycin.
(d) Clindamycin.
(e) Flucloxacillin.

Q24 Which of the following is the most useful test for determining the underlying organism in total joint replacements?

(a) Blood culture.
(b) Tissue culture.
(c) Wound swab.
(d) Joint aspirate culture.
(e) Urine sample culture.

(Q25) Which of the following factors does *not* increase the risk of thromboembolism?

(a) Smoking.
(b) General anaesthesia.
(c) Epidural anaesthesia.
(d) Obesity.
(e) Varicose veins.

(Q26) Which of the following anticoagulation agents relies on potentiation of antithrombin III action?

(a) Aspirin.
(b) Warfarin.
(c) Clopidogrel.
(d) Dextran.
(e) Heparin.

(Q27) What is the incidence of fatal pulmonary embolism after total hip replacement without the use of chemical prophylaxis?

(a) Less than 0.15%.
(b) Less than 0.35%.
(c) Less than 0.5%.
(d) Less than 1%.
(e) Less than 2%.

(Q28) A 39-year-old man is admitted to hospital having sustained bilateral femoral fractures. He is treated with bilateral intramedullary nails. Around 48 hours after injury he develops confusion, tachycardia, tachypnoea and a petechial rash. Which of the following is the most likely diagnosis?

(a) Pulmonary infection.
(b) Myocardial infarction.
(c) Fluid overload.
(d) Fat embolism.
(e) Pneumothorax.

Which of the following complications is *not* associated with blood transfusion?

(a)   HIV transmission.
(b)   Hypercalcaemia.
(c)   Hyperkalaemia.
(d)   Haemolytic reaction.
(e)   Febrile reaction.

 Which of the following statements concerning magnetic resonance imaging is *not* true?

(a)   Fat appears bright on T1-weighted images.
(b)   Fluid appears bright on T2-weighted images.
(c)   MRI uses radio-frequency pulses on tissues in a magnetic field.
(d)   MRI is the most sensitive method for detecting early osteonecrosis.
(e)   MRI aligns nuclei with odd numbers of electrons parallel to a magnetic field.

Answers

 (e).

 (b).

Calcitonin inhibits the function of osteoclasts, thereby inhibiting bone resorption.

 (b).

Oxygen tension is low in the reserve zone and highest in the proliferative zone. Oxygen tension then progressively decreases in the lower zones of the physis before increasing again in the metaphysis.

(a).

Cancellous bone provides an osteoconductive matrix into which bone growth can occur. It also contains osteoinductive factors which stimulate osteogenic cells to become activated and proliferate.

 (c).

Osteoporosis is a quantitative defect of bone, in which there is an overall reduction in bone mass. However, the proportion of mineralised bone remains normal. Osteomalacia and rickets are qualitative defects, in which overall bone mass may decline slightly, but the main abnormality is an increase in the proportion of unmineralised matrix.

A6 (e).

7-Dehydrocholesterol under the skin is converted to cholecalciferol by the action of sunlight. Cholecalciferol is also present in the normal diet, and undergoes 25-hydroxylation in the liver. 25-OH-cholecalciferol then undergoes 1-α-hydroxylation in the kidney to form 1,25-$(OH)_2$ cholecalciferol, the active metabolite of vitamin D.

A7 (a).

A8 (b).

A9 (a).

Approximately 50% of compressive strain is resisted by the superficial zone. Interstitial fluid exudation and tissue consolidation contribute to this property.

A10 (d).

The others are all mechanisms of lubrication, but elastohydrodynamic lubrication is the most important mechanism during joint movement.

A11 (c).

(A12)   (b).

Cartilage affected by osteoarthritis has an increased water content. This differs from degeneration that occurs in others tissues, such as tendon and intervertebral disc, where the water content decreases.

(A13)   (e).

Muscle contraction is triggered by an action potential travelling down a nerve. On reaching the neuromuscular junction, acetylcholine is released, which travels across the synaptic cleft and depolarises the muscle membrane. Subsequent depolarisation of the sarcoplasmic reticulum results in calcium release. Calcium binds to troponin, which is attached to actin. This results in a conformational change altering the position of tropomycin, which exposes actin and allows actin–myosin cross-bridges to be formed. Energy for this sliding filament mechanism is provided by the breakdown of ATP.

(A14)   (d).

The other signs are seen with upper motor neuron lesions.

(A15)   (a).

Neuropraxia is a transient, reversible block to nerve conduction. Axonotmesis occurs when the axon and myelin sheath are disrupted but the epineurium is intact. Neurotmesis is a complete division of a nerve fibre. Wallerian degeneration results in breakdown of myelin and occurs as a result of nerve injury. Epineurolysis is a surgical technique of dividing the epineurium in an attempt to relieve compression of nerves.

(A16)   (c).

This is the weakest point in the muscle-tendon subunit and the commonest site of rupture.

(A17)   (b).

IgM is the first immunoglobulin to increase in response to an acute infection. This is followed by a more important increase in IgG. IgA plays a role in protecting mucosal surfaces, and IgE is involved in allergic reactions. The role of IgD is poorly understood. However, it may play a role in modulating B-lymphocyte function.

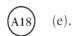 (e).

This observation has been made by several authors. Two recent examples are listed below.

- Pilcher J, Sogard L. Myelomeningocele, avocados, and rubber tree plants. *Neonatal Netw.* 2005; **24**: 23–8.
- Rendeli C *et al*. Latex sensitisation and allergy in children with myelomeningocele. *Childs Nerv Syst.* 2006; **22**: 28–32.

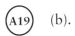 (b).

Staphylococcus aureus is the most important pathogen in orthopaedic practice. It is the most commonly implicated organism in surgical wound infections, osteomyelitis and septic arthritis.

(A20)   (d).

The proximal femoral metaphysis lies within the joint capsule of the hip joint. As a result, foci of osteomyelitis can disseminate into the joint, causing septic arthritis.

(A21)   (a).

The Working Party of the British Society of Antibacterial Chemotherapy has advised that no routine antibiotic prophylaxis is required for patients with prosthetic joints *in situ* who are undergoing dental work. However, many orthopaedic surgeons continue to advise the use of prophylactic antibiotics in such circumstances.

(A22)   (e).

 (d).

Although clindamycin reaches high concentrations in bone, its use is associated with a high incidence of pseudomembranous colitis. It should therefore be used judiciously.

 (b).

Tissue culture is the most accurate test for diagnosing infections in total joint replacements, but such samples can only be obtained surgically. Although other test samples are easier to obtain, they are not as reliable and can give rise to false-positive results.

 (c).

There is evidence that epidural anaesthesia helps to reduce the incidence of thromboembolism, by allowing earlier rehabilitation and by its sympatholytic action, which reduces venous stasis.

- Farag E *et al.* Epidural analgesia improves early rehabilitation after total knee replacement. *J Clin Anesth.* 2005; **17**: 281–5.
- Delis KT *et al.* Effects of epidural-and-general anesthesia combined versus general anesthesia alone on the venous hemodynamics of the lower limb. A randomised study. *Thromb Haemost.* 2004; **92**: 1003–11.

 (e).

Aspirin and clopidogrel inhibit platelet aggregation. Dextran works by diluting coagulation factors present in blood. Warfarin inhibits the vitamin K dependent factors II, VII, IX and X. Heparin exerts its action by potentiation of antithrombin III.

 (b).

There is an incidence of 70–80% for deep vein thrombosis diagnosed by venography following hip and knee replacement. However, the incidence of clinically significant deep vein thrombosis is much lower, at only 1–2%. The incidence of fatal pulmonary embolism after total hip replacement is very low, at only 0.34%.

- Warwick D *et al.* Death and thromboembolic disease after total hip replacement. A series of 1162 cases with no routine chemical prophylaxis. *J Bone Joint Surg Br.* 1995; **77**: 6–10.

(d).

Fat embolism occurs 24–72 hours after trauma. It is most commonly associated with long bone fractures, occurring in 3–4% of such cases. The fatality rate is 10–15%. The incidence of fat embolism can be reduced by early skeletal stabilisation of fractures. Confusion, tachycardia, tachypnoea and a petechial rash are typical clinical findings. Respiratory function gradually declines secondary to increased pulmonary capillary permeability, bronchoconstriction and alveolar collapse, resulting in a ventilation–perfusion mismatch consistent with adult respiratory distress syndrome (ARDS).

 (b).

Hypocalcaemia can result from blood transfusion.

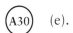 (e).

Nuclei with odd numbers of protons are aligned parallel to a magnetic field in magnetic resonance imaging.

Section 2

Biomechanics

(Q1) In relation to biomaterials, which of the following is a definition of stress?

(a) A measure of internal force.
(b) A measure of deformation.
(c) A measure of stiffness.
(d) A measure of energy.
(e) A measure of rigidity.

(Q2) On a stress–strain curve, which of the following is a definition of the yield point?

(a) The initial point at which the material begins to deform.
(b) The maximum strength achieved by the material.
(c) The transition point from elastic to plastic deformation.
(d) The point where the material fractures.
(e) The point at which viscoelastic deformation occurs.

(Q3) Which of the following terms describes materials that are able to undergo a large amount of plastic deformation prior to failure?

(a) Brittle.
(b) Viscoelastic.
(c) Anisotropic.
(d) Isotropic.
(e) Ductile.

Q4 Which of the following biomaterials is most likely to undergo pitting and crevice corrosion?

(a) Cobalt–chromium–molybdenum alloy.
(b) Stainless steel.
(c) Titanium.
(d) Polyethylene.
(e) Polymethylmethacrylate.

Q5 As which of the following is corrosion that occurs as a result of electrochemical destruction between dissimilar metals classified?

(a) Crevice.
(b) Galvanic.
(c) Fretting.
(d) Stress.
(e) Inclusional.

Q6 Which of the following materials has the highest stiffness?

(a) Bone.
(b) Tendon.
(c) Titanium.
(d) Ceramics.
(e) Stainless steel.

Q7 Which of the following statements about titanium is *not* true?

(a) Titanium has poor resistance to wear.
(b) Titanium particles may incite a histiocytic response.
(c) Titanium alloy generates less wear debris than cobalt–chrome alloy when used in total hip replacement prostheses.
(d) Titanium has a high yield strength.
(e) Titanium undergoes self-passivation to form an adherent oxide coating.

Which of the following statements relating to polyethylene is *not* true?

(a) Polyethylene displays viscoelastic properties.
(b) Polyethylene displays thermoplastic properties.
(c) Polyethylene generates free radicals in response to gamma irradiation.
(d) Polyethylene wear damage is most often the result of third-body inclusions.
(e) Polyethylene wear debris has no effect on the longevity of total hip replacements.

 Which of the following statements relating to bone cement (polymethylmethacrylate) is *not* true?

(a) Cement functions as an adhesive between bone and implants.
(b) Cement has poor tensile and shear strength.
(c) Polymerisation of cement is an exothermic reaction that occurs in three stages.
(d) Insertion of cement can lead to a significant drop in blood pressure.
(e) Reduction of the number of pores in cement can increase tensile strength.

 What is the reason for adding barium sulphate to bone cement?

(a) It acts as an accelerator.
(b) It acts as an inhibitor.
(c) It acts as a colouring agent.
(d) It acts as a radio-opacifier.
(e) It reduces cement wear debris.

 Which of the following properties do ceramic materials such as aluminium oxide (Al_2O_3) have?

(a) Low compressive strength.
(b) Low modulus of elasticity.

(c) Poor wear characteristics.
(d) Low fracture resistance.
(e) Low conductiveness to tissue bonding.

Q12 Which of the following statements about the mechanical properties of bone is *not* true?

(a) Bone is strongest in compression.
(b) The mineral content of bone is the main determinant of stiffness.
(c) Ageing results in a decrease in the cortical diameter of bone.
(d) Implants may lead to osteoporosis of adjacent bone.
(e) Bone is anisotropic and viscoelastic.

Q13 Which of the following statements about the mechanical properties of tendons is true?

(a) Ruptured tendons show histological evidence of inflammation.
(b) Ruptured tendons show histological evidence of degeneration.
(c) Tendons are strongest in compression.
(d) Tendons consist mainly of type II collagen.
(e) Tendons can withstand up to 25% strain prior to rupture.

Q14 Which of the following statements is true regarding the use of metal plates for internal fixation?

(a) Plates are load-sharing devices.
(b) A neutralisation plate applies static compression across a fracture.
(c) Plates are most effective when applied to the compression side of bone.
(d) Plate and screw removal after fracture union does not weaken the bone.
(e) Doubling the thickness of a plate increases rigidity by eightfold.

Q15 Which of the following statements is true regarding the use of intramedullary nails?

(a) Doubling the radius of an intramedullary nail increases rigidity by eightfold.
(b) Intramedullary nails are load-bearing devices.
(c) Intramedullary nails resist bending forces better than rotational forces.
(d) Material properties do not influence the rigidity of an intramedullary nail.
(e) There is no difference in torsional stiffness between closed-section and slotted nails.

 Q16 When using an external fixator, which of the following factors is most important for stability?

(a) Anatomical reduction of the fracture.
(b) Use of large-diameter pins.
(c) Decreased bone–rod distance.
(d) Using rods and pins in different planes.
(e) A near–near and far–far pin configuration in relation to the fracture site.

 Q17 Which of the following statements about total hip replacement is correct?

(a) The femoral stem should be placed in slight varus.
(b) Increasing the femoral component offset reduces the abductor moment arm.
(c) A smaller head size increases range of motion and stability.
(d) A large head size increases friction and volumetric polyethylene wear.
(e) The wear rate of ultra-high-molecular-weight polyethylene in the acetabulum is about 1 mm per year.

Q18   Which of the following measures does *not* help to optimise patellar tracking during total knee replacement?

(a)   Medial placement of the femoral component.
(b)   Lateral placement of the tibial component.
(c)   Medial placement of the patellar component.
(d)   Slight external rotation of the femoral component.
(e)   Avoiding malrotation of the tibial component.

Q19   Which of the following factors is most important in determining the joint reaction force?

(a)   Joint congruence.
(b)   Joint lubrication.
(c)   Joint contact area.
(d)   The muscles acting about a joint.
(e)   Articular cartilage thickness.

Q20   What is the optimal position for arthrodesis of the hip?

(a)   10° of flexion and 25° of abduction.
(b)   25° of flexion and 0° of abduction.
(c)   0° of flexion and 25° of abduction.
(d)   0° of flexion and 0° of abduction.
(e)   10° of extension and 25° of abduction.

Q21   Which of the following statements about movements of the knee joint is correct?

(a)   A normal knee cannot achieve any recurvatum.
(b)   The centre of rotation remains constant throughout the range of motion.
(c)   The femur externally rotates during the last 15° of extension.
(d)   The patella helps to increase the power of extension.
(e)   The anterior cruciate ligament controls femoral roll-back.

(Q22) Which of the following defines the mechanical axis of the lower limb?

(a) A line drawn from the centre of gravity to the ground.
(b) A line drawn from the centre of the femoral head to the centre of the knee.
(c) A line drawn from the centre of the femoral head to the centre of the ankle.
(d) A line drawn along the shaft of the femur and the tibia.
(e) A line drawn along the centre of the tibial plateau to the centre of the ankle.

(Q23) In relation to the mechanical axis of the lower limb, in which of the following is the anatomical axis of the femur?

(a) 3° of varus.
(b) 6° of varus.
(c) 0°.
(d) 3° of valgus.
(e) 6° of valgus.

(Q24) Which metatarsal bears the most weight during gait?

(a) First.
(b) Second.
(c) Third.
(d) Fourth.
(e) Fifth.

(Q25) What amount of shoulder abduction is achieved by glenohumeral movement?

(a) 30°.
(b) 60°.
(c) 90°.
(d) 120°.
(e) 150°.

Answers

A1   (a).

Stress is a measure of internal force and is calculated by the equation force/area.

A2   (c).

Once a material passes the yield point, it no longer displays elastic behaviour, and any deformation that occurs is not reversible.

A3   (e).

Ductile materials are able to undergo a large amount of plastic deformation, in contrast to brittle materials, which fail after relatively little plastic deformation. For viscoelastic materials, deformation depends on the load and its rate of application. Viscoelastic materials behave more elastically the more rapidly a load is applied. Isotropic materials have the same material properties in all directions. Anisotropic materials, such as bone, behave differently depending on the direction of loading.

A4   (b).

The area between the screw heads and the countersunk holes in stainless steel plates is a common site for crevice corrosion. Concerns about corrosion of stainless steel implants have relegated their use to temporary devices such as fracture fixation plates.

A5   (b).

The risk of galvanic corrosion is highest between 316L stainless steel and cobalt–chromium alloy. In total joint replacements, modular components have direct contact. Therefore it is important not to use components made from different metals.

A6   (d).

Ceramics are solid compounds, consisting of organic and inorganic materials. They are very hard, stiff and brittle. They are very strong under compressive loads, have very low wear rates and are highly biocompatible. These properties make them ideal for use in orthopaedic implants.

 (c).

Although titanium is able to undergo self-passivation, which reduces wear, it still has poor wear resistance. The generated wear particles can incite a histiocytic response.

 (e).

Polyethylene wear debris is the most important factor affecting the longevity of total joint replacements.

 (a).

Polymethylmethacrylate cement functions as a grout by mechanically interlocking with bone. The polymerisation process occurs in three stages consisting of initiation, propagation and termination. Reduction of pores in cement, which can be achieved by vacuum mixing, reduces the incidence of cracks and increases tensile strength.

 (d).

Agents such as barium sulphate and zirconium dioxide are commonly added to bone cement as radio-opacifiers to aid radiological diagnosis.

 (d).

Ceramics are very hard, stiff and strong under compressive loads, but they are brittle, which makes them susceptible to fracture. There have been many reports in the literature of fracture of total hip replacement components.

- Habermann *et al.* Fracture of ceramic heads in total hip replacement. *Arch Orthop Trauma Surg.* 2006; **126**: 464–70.

(A12) (c).

With ageing, the material properties of bone decline. To compensate for this, the inner and outer cortical diameters of bone increase. When orthopaedic implants are inserted, adjacent areas of bone are deprived of normal physiological loading, which results in localised osteoporosis. This phenomenon is known as stress shielding.

(A13) (b).

Tendon rupture is unlikely to occur in healthy tendons. Most tendons that rupture have pre-existing degenerative changes. The following papers support this observation.

- Kannus P, Jozsa L. Histopathological changes preceding spontaneous rupture of a tendon. A controlled study of 891 patients. *J Bone Joint Surg Am.* 1991; **73**: 1507–25.
- Sharma P, Maffulli N. Tendon injury and tendinopathy: healing and repair. *J Bone Joint Surg Am.* 2005; **87**: 187–202.

(A14) (e).

The rigidity of metal plates is proportional to the cube value of the thickness (t^3).

(A15) (c).

Doubling the radius of a nail increases bending rigidity by 16-fold, as bending rigidity is proportional to the fourth power of the radius (r^4). Intramedullary nails are load-sharing devices. Material and structural properties clearly affect the mechanical properties of a nail, and closed-section nails have a higher torsional stiffness than slotted nails.

(A16) (a).

Anatomical reduction is the most important factor in determining stability when applying an external fixator. The second most important factor is the use of large-diameter pins, as the bending rigidity of pins is proportional to the fourth power of the radius (r^4).

(A17) (d).

Although large head sizes improve range of motion and stability, they increase friction and volumetric wear of polyethylene. Smaller head sizes lead to less polyethylene wear, but are not as stable and permit a smaller range of motion. Therefore the choice of head size needs to be a compromise between these two extremes, and is often 26 or 28 mm. The wear rate of ultra-high-molecular-weight poly-ethylene in the acetabulum is about 0.1 mm per year.

 (a).

Medial placement of the femoral component will predispose to lateral subluxation of the patella. In order to avoid such mal-tracking, the femoral component should be placed laterally, whilst the patellar component is positioned medially.

 (d).

The most important determinant of joint reaction force is the muscles acting about a joint. This is the mechanism of action of many orthopaedic orthotic devices. Orthoses stabilise a joint by eliminating the movement of muscles around the joint. The sub-sequent reduction in joint reaction force offloads the joint and results in pain relief.

 (b).

In arthrodesis of the hip it is important to avoid any abduction. If the hip is placed in an abducted position, the patient tends to lurch over the affected limb, resulting in lower back pain.

 (d).

The patella helps to increase the power of extension. Patellectomy reduces the moment arm for extension by the width of the patella. This has been estimated to result in a 30% loss of power of extension.

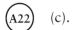 (c).

(a) is the vertical axis, (b) is the mechanical axis of the femur, (c) represents the mechanical axis of the lower limb, (d) represents the anatomic axes of the femur and tibia, and (e) is the mechanical axis of the tibia.

 (e).

A24 (b).

During stance the first metatarsal bears the most weight. However, during gait it is the second metatarsal which takes most of the weight.

A25 (d).

The 180° of shoulder abduction is made up of glenohumeral (120°) and scapulothoracic (60°) motion in a 2:1 ratio.

Section 3

Paediatric orthopaedics

Q1 A 1-week-old baby is noted to have a swelling superior to the left clavicle. The baby is also noted to have left metatarsus adductus. Which of the following is the most likely diagnosis of the swelling?

(a) Shoulder dislocation/dystocia.
(b) Sprengel's deformity.
(c) Congenital muscular torticollis.
(d) Congenital pseudarthrosis of the clavicle.
(e) Cervical rib.

Q2 A 2-year-old child who has cerebral palsy can only abduct his hip to 25°. Radiographs demonstrate 40% uncovering of the femoral head. Which of the following is the most appropriate management?

(a) Abduction bracing.
(b) Femoral osteotomy.
(c) Pelvic osteotomy.
(d) Adductor tenotomy.
(e) Any surgery should be delayed until the child is 3 years old.

Q3 Which of the following shows a reduction in incidence if there is maternal supplementation of folic acid?

(a) Myelomeningocoele.
(b) Arthrogryposis.
(c) Muscular dystrophy.

   (d)   Peroneal muscular atrophy.
   (e)   Myasthenia gravis.

Q4   A 12-year-old girl presents with kyphoscoliosis of her lumbar spine. She is noted to have multiple light brown spots on her skin, and slit-lamp examination reveals lesions in her iris. What is her underlying diagnosis?

   (a)   Friedreich's ataxia.
   (b)   Scheuermann's disease.
   (c)   Idiopathic scoliosis.
   (d)   Marfan's syndrome.
   (e)   Neurofibromatosis.

Q5   What is the most common type of deformity seen in scoliosis?

   (a)   Left thoracic.
   (b)   Right thoracic.
   (c)   Double major.
   (d)   Left lumbar.
   (e)   Right lumbar.

Q6   Which type of scoliosis curve must always be evaluated with an MRI scan?

   (a)   Left thoracic.
   (b)   Right thoracic.
   (c)   Double major.
   (d)   Left lumbar.
   (e)   Right lumbar.

Q7   In children undergoing posterior spinal fusion for scoliosis correction, the crankshaft phenomenon occurs secondary to which of the following?

   (a)   Development of a pseudarthrosis.
   (b)   Implant failure.
   (c)   Deformity overcorrection.

(d) Infection.

(e) Continued anterior spinal growth.

Q8 An increased incidence of late-onset low back pain is seen after spinal fusion for scoliosis, if the fusion extends below which of the following levels?

(a) L1.

(b) L2.

(c) L3.

(d) L4.

(e) L5.

Q9 In congenital scoliosis, with which of the following is the risk of curve progression highest?

(a) Unsegmented hemivertebra.

(b) Incarcerated hemivertebra.

(c) Unilateral unsegmented bar.

(d) Unilateral unsegmented bar with contralateral hemi-vertebra.

(e) Fully segmented hemivertebra.

Q10 A 6-month-old girl was noted to have spastic paraplegia of the lower limbs and poor anal sphincter tone. An MRI scan demonstrated an osseous bar creating a longitudinal cleft in the spinal cord. What is the most likely underlying diagnosis?

(a) Meningocoele.

(b) Myelomeningocoele.

(c) Spina bifida cystica.

(d) Diastomatomyelia.

(e) Spina bifida occulta.

Q11 A 15-year-old cricket player presents with a 6-month history of lower back pain. No associated neurological symptoms are present. His blood test results are normal. Radiographs appear normal apart from slight anterior translation of L5 on the sacrum. Which of the following is the most likely diagnosis?

(a) Spina bifida occulta.
(b) Spondylolysis.
(c) Discitis.
(d) Sacral agenesis.
(e) Scheurmann's disease.

Q12 An 11-year-old girl presents with shoulder elevation and a rib rotation deformity. Her radiographs demonstrate a right-sided thoracic scoliosis. Which of the following is Risser staging used to determine?

(a) The type of curve.
(b) The neutral vertebra.
(c) The appropriate levels of fusion.
(d) The risk of curve progression.
(e) The skeletal maturity of the patient.

Q13 What is the commonest cause of intoeing gait in young children?

(a) Tibial torsion.
(b) Femoral retroversion.
(c) Metatarsus adductus.
(d) Skew foot.
(e) Rickets.

Q14 With which of the following conditions is metatarsus adductus commonly associated?

(a) Tarsal coalition.
(b) Proximal femoral focal deficiency.
(c) Developmental dysplasia of the hip.

    (d)   Perthes' disease.
    (e)   Blount's disease.

Q15 Which of the following is *not* associated with an increased risk of developmental dysplasia of the hip?

    (a)   Female sex.
    (b)   Breech delivery.
    (c)   Positive family history.
    (d)   Congenital muscular torticollis.
    (e)   Decreased maternal oestrogen.

Q16 When assessing an AP pelvis radiograph for developmental dysplasia of the hip, which of the following is the term for a line passing through the triradiate cartilages?

    (a)   Shenton's line.
    (b)   Perkin's line.
    (c)   Klein's line.
    (d)   Hilgenreiner's line.
    (e)   Trethowan's line.

Q17 A 4-month-old girl is referred to the orthopaedic clinic. Her mother is concerned about a clicking left hip. Clinically Ortolani's test is positive, and the child's radiographs support a diagnosis of developmental dysplasia of the hip. Which of the following is the most appropriate form of management?

    (a)   Application of a Pavlik harness.
    (b)   Application of a hip spica.
    (c)   Closed reduction and application of a Pavlik harness.
    (d)   Closed reduction and application of a hip spica.
    (e)   Open reduction.

Q18 Which of the following is the most important risk of reduction in developmental dysplasia of the hip?

(a) Failure to achieve a concentric reduction.
(b) Femoral nerve palsy.
(c) Recurrent dislocation.
(d) Avascular necrosis.
(e) Femoral fracture.

Q19 Which of the following is *not* associated with an increased risk of developing Perthes' disease of the hip?

(a) Male sex.
(b) Abnormal birth presentation.
(c) Low birth weight.
(d) Positive family history.
(e) Congenital muscular torticollis.

Q20 In Perthes' disease, which of the following is the process by which replacement of necrotic bone occurs?

(a) Appositional repair.
(b) Creeping substitution.
(c) Fragmentation.
(d) Reossification.
(e) Remodelling.

Q21 A 6-year-old boy who has Perthes' disease is found to have a crescent sign on his radiographs. What does the crescent sign represent?

(a) A fracture of necrotic bone.
(b) Lateral subluxation.
(c) Metaphyseal cyst formation.
(d) Remodelling.
(e) Reossification.

(Q22) Which of the following radiographic features is *not* one of Catterall's 'head at risk' signs?

(a) Gage's sign.
(b) The crescent sign.
(c) Lateral subluxation.
(d) Lateral calcification.
(e) Metaphyseal cyst formation.

(Q23) What is the incidence of bilateral involvement in slipped upper femoral epiphysis?

(a) 10%.
(b) 20%.
(c) 25%.
(d) 40%.
(e) 50%.

(Q24) Which of the following is the characteristic displacement in slipped upper femoral epiphysis?

(a) Anterior displacement of the femoral head.
(b) Lateral displacement of the femoral head.
(c) Medial displacement of the femoral head.
(d) Anterior displacement and external rotation of the femoral neck.
(e) Posterior displacement and internal rotation of the femoral neck.

(Q25) An obese 9-year-old boy presents to the emergency department complaining of a 1-day history of pain in his right hip and knee. Blood parameters are unremarkable. Radiographs show evidence of a right slipped upper femoral epiphysis. Which of the following conditions also needs to be excluded?

(a) Blount's disease.
(b) Haemophilia.
(c) Protein C deficiency.

(d) Metatarsus adductus.

(e) Hypothyroidism.

Q26 A 14-year-old boy presents to the emergency department with a 1-month history of left hip pain. Blood parameters are unremarkable. Radiographs show evidence of a grade II slip of the left upper femoral epiphysis. Which of the following is the most appropriate form of management?

(a) Closed reduction and fixation with a single cannulated screw.

(b) Closed reduction and fixation with cannulated screws in a triangular formation.

(c) Open reduction and internal fixation.

(d) Fixation *in situ* with a single cannulated screw.

(e) Fixation *in situ* with cannulated screws in a triangular formation.

Q27 A 15-year-old girl is seen in the outpatient clinic 3 months after surgery for a slipped right upper femoral epiphysis. Over the last month she has noticed increased discomfort in her right hip. Review of her notes reveals that surgery was technically difficult and several passes of the guide wire were required to obtain satisfactory position. Fluoroscopy films reveal an episode of intra-articular guide-wire penetration. Which of the following is the most likely underlying diagnosis?

(a) Septic arthritis of the hip.

(b) Chondrolysis.

(c) Avascular necrosis.

(d) Fixation failure.

(e) Flexion contracture of the hip.

An 8-year-old boy is brought to the emergency department by his parents. He has been limping for the past 2 days, and is now unable to bear weight. He complains of pain in his right groin and knee. He is pyrexial with a temperature of 39°. Blood tests reveal a WBC of 15.4 x 10^9 and an ESR of 78 mm/hour. Which of the following is the most likely diagnosis?

(a) Septic arthritis of the hip.
(b) Perthes' disease.
(c) Slipped upper femoral epiphysis.
(d) Developmental dysplasia of the hip.
(e) Transient synovitis of the hip.

 In which area does osteomyelitis usually begin in children?

(a) The joint.
(b) The epiphysis.
(c) The physis.
(d) The metaphysis.
(e) The diaphysis.

 A 4-year-old boy of Afro-Caribbean origin is seen in the outpatient clinic. His parents complain that his legs are bowed out. He is not known to have any medical problems. Radiographs demonstrate irregularity at the medial proximal tibial physis with metaphyseal beaking. Which of the following is the most likely cause of his bowed legs?

(a) Osteogenesis imperfecta.
(b) Rickets.
(c) Blount's disease.
(d) Osteochondroma.
(e) Normal physiological bowing.

Q31 In which of the following conditions is parallelism and loss of talocalcaneal divergence seen on radiographs?

(a) Skew foot.
(b) Metatarsus adductus.
(c) Pes cavus.
(d) Congenital vertical talus.
(e) Congenital talipes equinovarus.

Q32 Which of the following conditions is the most commonly seen congenital orthopaedic anomaly?

(a) Congenital talipes equinovarus.
(b) Congenital vertical talus.
(c) Fibular hemimelia.
(d) Tibial hemimelia.
(e) Ball-and-socket ankle.

Q33 A 6-year-old girl was seen in the emergency department after having fallen and sustained a supracondylar fracture of her right humerus. On examination she was unable to touch the tips of her right thumb and index finger together. Sensation was found to be normal and no other motor deficit was present. Involvement of which of the following nerves would account for these findings?

(a) Posterior interosseous nerve.
(b) Anterior interosseous nerve.
(c) Radial nerve.
(d) Ulnar nerve.
(e) Musculocutaneous nerve.

Q34 A 7-year-old boy is admitted to hospital after sustaining a supracondylar fracture of his right humerus. He is taken to theatre and a closed reduction is performed, followed by insertion of crossed K-wires. After recovery from surgery, he is found to have diminished sensation in his right ring and little fingers and is unable to abduct his fingers. Injury of which of the following nerves would account for the clinical findings?

(a) Posterior interosseous nerve.
(b) Anterior interosseous nerve.
(c) Radial nerve.
(d) Ulnar nerve.
(e) Musculocutaneous nerve.

(Q35) On evaluation of lateral radiographs of the elbow, what is the value of the humero-condylar angle?

(a) 10°.
(b) 20°.
(c) 30°.
(d) 40°.
(e) 50°.

(Q36) A 5-year-old boy was brought to the emergency department after falling off his bicycle and banging his head. Initially he complained of some pain in his neck, and radiographs of his cervical spine were taken. The radiographs showed slight anterior translation of C2 on C3. This was measured to be 3 mm. The posterior spinolaminar line was well aligned and no soft tissue swelling was noted. By the time he was examined, his neck pain had resolved and no neurological deficit was present. What is the most likely diagnosis?

(a) SCIWORA.
(b) Odontoid peg fracture.
(c) Pseudosubluxation.
(d) Unilateral facet joint dislocation.
(e) Hangman fracture.

(Q37) With regard to femoral shaft fractures, which of the following types of displacement has the poorest remodelling potential?

(a) Varus angulation.
(b) Valgus angulation.

(c)   Shortening.
(d)   Lateral translation.
(e)   Rotation.

 Q38 According to the Salter and Harris classification of physeal injuries, how is a fracture that extends through the meta-physis, physis and epiphysis classified?

(a)   Type I.
(b)   Type II.
(c)   Type III.
(d)   Type IV.
(e)   Type V.

 Q39 A 13-year-old boy has sustained a three-part triplane frac-ture of his left ankle. According to the Salter and Harris classification of physeal injuries, what type of fracture will be seen on lateral radiographs?

(a)   Type I.
(b)   Type II.
(c)   Type III.
(d)   Type IV.
(e)   Type V.

 Q40 Which of the following fractures would be most likely to alert a physician to the possibility of non-accidental injury?

(a)   Middle third clavicle fracture.
(b)   Spiral fracture of the tibia.
(c)   Linear skull fracture.
(d)   Salter Harris II distal radius fracture.
(e)   Distal femoral metaphysis corner fracture.

Answers

 (c).

There is an association between congenital muscular torticollis and other 'packaging disorders' such as metatarsus adductus and developmental dysplasia of the hip.

 (d).

In general, surgery should be avoided in the first 3 years in children suffering from cerebral palsy. However, if hip abduction is less than 45° and radiographs demonstrate partial uncovering of the femoral head, the hip is deemed to be at risk. This is the only situation in which surgery is indicated below the age of 3 years, and an adductor tenotomy with or without a psoas release is the operation of choice.

 (a).

Periconceptional maternal folic acid supplementation reduces the incidence of neural-tube defects. Such supplementation has resulted in a 25–30% reduction in the incidence of neural-tube defects.

- Pitkin RM. Folate and neural tube defects. *Am J Clin Nutr.* 2007; **85**: 285–8S.

 (e).

Neurofibromatosis, an autosomal dominant disorder of neural crest origin, can result in neuromuscular scoliosis. Diagnostic criteria include affected first-degree relative, at least six café-au-lait spots, two or more neurofibromas, multiple axillary or inguinal freckles, osseous lesions, optic gliomas, and two or more iris lesions seen on slit-lamp examination (Lish nodules). At least two of the above criteria are required to establish a diagnosis.

 (b).

(A6)   (a).

There is a high incidence of intraspinal anomalies such as syringo-myelia associated with such curves. Therefore magnetic resonance imaging is mandatory.

(A7)   (e).

The crankshaft phenomenon occurs secondary to posterior spinal fusion in skeletally immature patients, which prevents posterior spinal growth but allows continued anterior spinal growth. Increased spinal rotation and deformity occur.

(A8)   (c).

There is a marked increase with fusion to L5 and some increase with fusion to L4. Therefore every effort should be made to stop fusion at L3.

(A9)   (d).

(A10)   (d).

Diastomatomyelia is a condition that leads to splitting of the spinal cord, resulting in the formation of two hemicords. An osseous, fibrous or cartilaginous bar splits the spinal cord, creating a longi-tudinal cleft. It usually occurs in the lumbar spine, and inter-pedicular widening seen on plain radiographs is suggestive of the diagnosis. Spina bifida occulta is a defect in the vertebral arch without protrusion of the cord or its membranes. Spina bifida cystica includes conditions such as meningocoele and myelomeningocoele, in which there is protrusion of the spinal membranes alone and the spinal membranes together with spinal cord, respectively.

(A11)   (b).

Spondylolysis is common in young adolescents who are involved in athletic activities that cause hyperextension of the spine. The underlying cause of the spondylolysis is a stress fracture of the pars interarticularis.

(e).

Risser staging is a technique for determining skeletal maturity by assessing iliac apophysis ossification. Ossification commences at the anterior superior iliac spine and progresses posteromedially. The iliac crest is divided into quadrants, so when 50% is ossified it is Risser stage 2. Risser stage 5 is reached when all of the quadrants are ossified and the apophysis is fused to the iliac crest.

 (a).

Tibial torsion is the commonest cause of an intoeing gait. It is thought to result from abnormal intrauterine positioning, and is associated with other 'packaging disorders' such as metatarsus adductus. Tibial torsion typically presents in the second year of life, and is often bilateral. Spontaneous resolution usually occurs, and surgical intervention is rarely required.

 (c).

There is an association between metatarsus adductus and developmental dysplasia of the hip.

- Kumar SJ, MacEwen GD. The incidence of hip dysplasia with metatarsus adductus. *Clin Orthop Relat Res.* 1982; **164**: 234–5.

 (e).

Decreased maternal oestrogen does not increase the risk of developmental dysplasia of the hip, although there is some evidence from animal studies that increased levels may play a role.

 (d).

Shenton's line is formed by the superior aspect of the obturator foramen and the medial aspect of the femoral neck. This line is broken in femoral neck fractures and hip subluxation or dislocation. Perkin's line is drawn perpendicular to Hilgenreiner's line at the lateral edge of the acetabulum. Ideally this line should bisect the femoral shaft and the femoral head should lie medial to it. Klein's line and Trethowan's line are different names for a line drawn along the superior border of the femoral neck to assess for slipped upper femoral epiphysis.

 (c).

In newborns and infants up to 6 months of age, closed reduction and immobilisation in a Pavlik harness is the treatment of choice. After application of the harness, radiographs or an ultrasound scan should be obtained to demonstrate satisfactory reduction. Stability of the reduction must also be demonstrated by obtaining imaging 2–4 weeks after harness application.

 (d).

Avascular necrosis can be seen with all forms of treatment for developmental dysplasia of the hip. Causes include extrinsic compression of the vasculature supplying the capital femoral epiphysis, and excessive direct pressure on the cartilaginous femoral head. Excessive or forceful abduction is also a risk factor, and extreme positions of abduction should be avoided.

(A19) (e).

Congenital muscular torticollis is associated with developmental dysplasia of the hip, but not with Perthes' disease.

(A20) (b).

Creeping substitution is the process by which necrotic bone is removed as a result of osteoclastic resorption. New vascular channels are formed and osteoblasts then lay down new bone, resulting in the formation of new Haversian systems.

(A21) (a).

The crescent sign represents a fracture of necrotic subchondral bone.

(A22) (b).

Catterall's 'head at risk' signs are associated with a poor prognosis in Perthes' disease. Although the crescent sign is often seen on radiographs in Perthes' disease, it is not one of Catterall's 'head at risk' signs.

 (c).

The incidence of bilateral involvement in slipped upper femoral epiphysis is up to 25%. It is believed to be even higher in patients with an endocrinopathy, and prophylactic fixation is advised in these patients.

 (d).

The head actually remains *in situ* and the femoral neck displaces anteriorly and externally rotates. On plain radiographs this gives the impression that the head has fallen off the back.

(A25)   (e).

There is an increased incidence of slipped upper femoral epiphysis in children suffering from hypothyroidism.

- Puri R *et al.* Slipped upper femoral epiphysis and primary juvenile hypothyroidism. *J Bone Joint Surg Br.* 1985; **67**: 14–20.

(A26)   (d).

Currently accepted practice is to fix the slipped epiphysis *in situ* with a single screw. It has been suggested that reduction can result in an increased incidence of avascular necrosis, although some authors have reported that acute reduction within 24 hours is not associated with such complications.

(A27)   (b).

Intra-articular penetration of guide wires or screws is associated with an increased risk of developing chondrolysis.

- Vrettos BC, Hoffman EB. Chondrolysis in slipped upper femoral epiphysis. Long-term study of the aetiology and natural history. *J Bone Joint Surg Br.* 1993; **75**: 956–61.

(A28)   (a).

Four important parameters have been identified in diagnosing septic arthritis of the hip, namely inability to weight bear, history of fever, a white cell count of $> 12 \times 10^9$, and an erythrocyte sedimentation rate of > 40 mm/hour. If all four parameters are positive, as in this case, the predicted probability of septic arthritis is 99.6%.

- Kocher MS *et al.* Differentiating between septic arthritis and transient synovitis of the hip in children: an evidence-based clinical prediction algorithm. *J Bone Joint Surg Am.* 1999; **81:** 1662–70.

(A29)   (d).

In the metaphyseal sinusoids the blood flow is sluggish and oxygen tension is high. Consequently, the metaphysis is an ideal area for bacteria to multiply if seeding occurs.

(A30)   (c).

Blount's disease typically causes these clinical and radiographic features, and is more common in individuals of Afro-Caribbean origin.

(A31)   (e).

In congenital talipes equinovarus, parallelism between the talus and calcaneus is lost and the longitudinal axes of the two bones become divergent.

(A32)   (a).

The incidence of congenital talipes equinovarus is 1 in 1000.

(A33)   (b).

The anterior interosseous nerve arises from the median nerve 5 cm below the medial epicondyle, and is therefore at risk of injury in supracondylar fractures of the humerus. It supplies the flexor pollicis longus and the lateral half of the flexor digitorum profundus, but does not have any sensory cutaneous branches.

A34 (d).

Injury to the ulnar nerve would account for these clinical findings. The ulnar nerve runs behind the medial epicondyle, and is at risk of being injured when fixation wires are being inserted. Consequently, many surgeons advocate that a small incision should be made prior to insertion of medial wires in fixation of supracondylar humeral fractures.

A35 (d).

Evaluation of this angle is useful when assessing for supracondylar fractures of the humerus. In such cases the angle is generally increased, as most supracondylar fractures are extension type.

A36 (c).

Subluxation of C2 on C3, and occasionally of C3 on C4, of up to 40% or 4 mm is seen in children under 8 years of age. Lack of anterior neck swelling, continued alignment of the posterior spinolaminar line and reduction of subluxation with neck extension helps to distinguish this entity from serious injury.

A37 (e).

Rotation has the poorest remodelling potential and therefore should not be accepted, as it will result in long-term problems.

A38 (d).

A39 (b).

In three-part triplane fractures, the lateral radiograph demonstrates a type II fracture, and a type III fracture is seen on the AP view.

(e).

Metaphyseal corner fractures, also known as bucket-handle fractures, are almost pathognomonic of non-accidental injury. They should alert the physician to this possibility, and a thorough examination of the child should be performed, including a complete radiographic skeletal survey.

Section 4

Hip and femur

Q1 Which artery supplies blood to the femoral head via the ligamentum teres?

  (a) Medial circumflex femoral artery.
  (b) Lateral circumflex femoral artery.
  (c) Obturator artery.
  (d) Superior gluteal artery.
  (e) Inferior gluteal artery.

Q2 From which artery does the gluteus medius muscle receive its main blood supply?

  (a) Medial circumflex femoral artery.
  (b) Lateral circumflex femoral artery.
  (c) Obturator artery.
  (d) Superior gluteal artery.
  (e) Inferior gluteal artery.

Q3 What is the nerve supply of the piriformis muscle?

  (a) Superior gluteal nerve.
  (b) Inferior gluteal nerve.
  (c) Femoral nerve.
  (d) Obturator nerve.
  (e) First and second sacral nerves.

Q4 Pain originating from the hip joint is often referred to the knee joint. Which nerve is responsible for this finding?

  (a) Femoral nerve.
  (b) Obturator nerve.

(c)   Sciatic nerve.
(d)   Superior gluteal nerve.
(e)   Inferior gluteal nerve.

Q5   Where is the origin of the straight head of the rectus femoris?

(a)   Anterior inferior iliac spine.
(b)   Anterior superior iliac spine.
(c)   Ilium superior to the acetabulum.
(d)   Superior pubic ramus.
(e)   Proximal anterior femur.

Q6   Where is the insertion of the iliotibial tract?

(a)   Patella.
(b)   Lateral femoral condyle.
(c)   Tibial tubercle.
(d)   Fibular head.
(e)   Gerdy's tubercle.

Q7   Weakness of which muscle group is elicited by performing Trendelenberg's test?

(a)   Hip flexors.
(b)   Hip extensors.
(c)   Hip adductors.
(d)   Hip abductors.
(e)   Hip short external rotators.

Q8   Which of the following tests can be performed in order to elicit a fixed flexion deformity of the hip?

(a)   Trendelenberg's test.
(b)   Thomas's test.
(c)   Speed's test.
(d)   McMurray's test.
(e)   Froment's test.

Q9 When assessing AP radiographs of total hip replacements for loosening, how many DeLee and Charnley zones are present?

(a) 1.
(b) 2.
(c) 3.
(d) 4.
(e) 5.

Q10 An 84-year-old man complains of pain in his right hip, which was replaced 16 years ago. An AP radiograph shows evidence of loosening below the tip of the femoral component. Which Gruen zone does this correspond to?

(a) 3.
(b) 4.
(c) 7.
(d) 9.
(e) 12.

Q11 Which of the following parameters is the centre edge angle of Wiberg used to assess?

(a) Acetabular retroversion.
(b) Acetabular protrusion.
(c) Acetabular dysplasia.
(d) Femoro-acetabular impingement.
(e) Femoral anteversion.

Q12 What is the most frequently used method of polyethylene sterilisation?

(a) Gamma irradiation.
(b) Ethylene oxide gas.
(c) Glutaraldehyde.
(d) Autoclaving.
(e) 100% alcohol.

Q13 Which of the following is a feature of third-generation cementing technique?

(a) Femoral canal brushing.
(b) Cement gun.
(c) Pulse lavage.
(d) Cement restrictor.
(e) Vacuum mixing.

Q14 In total hip replacement surgery, by which of the following measures can the primary arc of movement be increased?

(a) Increasing acetabular component anteversion.
(b) Increasing femoral component anteversion.
(c) Insertion of a hooded acetabular liner.
(d) Increasing neck length.
(e) Increasing the diameter of the femoral head.

Q15 Which of the following complications is characteristically associated with metal-on-metal hip resurfacing arthroplasty?

(a) Dislocation.
(b) Pulmonary embolism.
(c) Avascular necrosis.
(d) Femoral neck fracture.
(e) Heterotopic ossification.

Q16 Which of the following complications has an increased incidence following total hip replacement in patients with Parkinson's disease?

(a) Pulmonary embolism.
(b) Heterotopic ossification.
(c) Dislocation.
(d) Myocardial infarction.
(e) Cerebrovascular accident.

Which nerve is most commonly injured during total hip replacement?

(a) Femoral nerve.
(b) Obturator nerve.
(c) Superior gluteal nerve.
(d) Inferior gluteal nerve.
(e) Sciatic nerve.

 A 27-year-old woman complains of a burning pain and numbness affecting the anterolateral part of her proximal right thigh. Her symptoms are reproduced by deep palpation just below the anterior superior iliac spine. What is the underlying diagnosis?

(a) Trochanteric bursitis.
(b) Meralgia paraesthetica.
(c) Avulsion of the origin of the sartorius.
(d) Anterior superior iliac spine osteomyelitis.
(e) Snapping hip syndrome.

 Which of the following abnormalities is characteristically seen in rheumatoid arthritis?

(a) Acetabular retroversion.
(b) Acetabular protrusion.
(c) Acetabular dysplasia.
(d) Reduced femoral offset.
(e) Femoral retroversion.

 Which of the following is *not* a risk factor for avascular necrosis of the femoral head?

(a) Steroids.
(b) Diuretics.
(c) Sickle-cell disease.
(d) Pregnancy.
(e) Radiotherapy.

Q21 Which of the following muscles results in external rotation of the affected limb in femoral neck fracture?

(a) Iliopsoas.
(b) Rectus femoris.
(c) Vastus lateralis.
(d) Adductor magnus.
(e) Gluteus maximus.

Q22 Which of the following is the most important predictor of fixation failure when using a dynamic hip screw?

(a) The extent of fracture comminution.
(b) The mental capacity of the patient.
(c) The tip–apex distance of the lag screw.
(d) The length of the plate.
(e) The angle of plate and screw.

Q23 When using a dynamic hip screw, with what screw length should a short barrel plate be used?

(a) 100 mm.
(b) 95 mm.
(c) 90 mm.
(d) 85 mm.
(e) 80 mm.

Q24 What is the most important predictor of functional outcome following proximal femoral fractures?

(a) The extent of fracture comminution.
(b) The method of fixation/replacement.
(c) Patient comorbidity.
(d) The mental capacity of the patient.
(e) The timing of surgery.

Q25 A 37-year-old motorcyclist presents to the emergency department after being involved in a road traffic accident. He has sustained a displaced femoral neck fracture. What is the most appropriate form of management?

(a) Total hip replacement.
(b) Reduction and internal fixation.
(c) Cemented Thompson hemiarthroplasty.
(d) Uncemented bipolar hemiarthroplasty.
(e) Intramedullary nailing.

Q26 With cannulated screw fixation of femoral neck fractures, with which of the following complications is an entry point below the lesser trochanter associated?

(a) Non-union.
(b) Avascular necrosis.
(c) Chondrolysis.
(d) Subtrochanteric fracture.
(e) Screw cutout.

Q27 Up to what percentage of non-union rates have been reported after internal fixation of displaced intracapsular femoral neck fractures?

(a) 10%.
(b) 20%.
(c) 30%.
(d) 40%.
(e) 50%.

Q28 What is the approximate amount of anteversion present in the femoral neck?

(a) 5°.
(b) 15°.
(c) 25°.
(d) 35°.
(e) 45°.

A 42-year-old woman gives a 6-month history of right hip pain. On examination she has reduced internal rotation, and hip flexion, internal rotation and adduction reproduce her pain. Radiographs show a congruent joint with adequate joint space. However, the femoral head:neck ratio is reduced. What is the cause of her hip pain?

(a) Femoroacetabular impingement.
(b) Osteoarthritis.
(c) Avascular necrosis.
(d) Adductor tendinopathy.
(e) Iliopsoas tendon rupture.

 Which of the following conditions is associated with pincer-type femoroacetabular impingement?

(a) Femoral anteversion.
(b) Femoral neck fracture malunion.
(c) Perthes' disease.
(d) Slipped upper femoral epiphysis.
(e) Acetabular retroversion.

Answers

 (c).

The obturator artery arises from the internal iliac artery. It gives a posterior branch to the acetabulum and then gives off a branch to the ligamentum teres, which supplies blood to the femoral head.

 (d).

The superior gluteal artery leaves the pelvis through the greater sciatic notch, where it passes above the piriformis tendon. It is the major blood supply to the gluteus minimus and medius. It also gives off a superficial branch which supplies the gluteus maximus.

 (e).

The piriformis muscle arises from the anterior aspect of the sacrum and passes through the greater sciatic notch to insert into the piriform fossa of the greater trochanter of the femur. It is supplied by the first and second sacral nerves.

 (b).

The obturator nerve arises from the anterior divisions of the L2,3,4 nerve roots. It passes through the pelvis and then enters the upper part of the obturator foramen, where it divides into its various branches.

 (a).

The rectus femoris muscle arises from two heads. The straight head originates from the anterior inferior iliac spine, and the reflected head arises from the ilium above the acetabulum. Distally it forms a common tendon along with the other muscles which make up the quadriceps, and inserts into the patella.

 (e).

The iliotibial tract is a downward continuation of the fascia lata. It is attached to the lateral condyle of the tibia, which is known as Gerdy's tubercle. The iliotibial tract helps to maintain the knee in a hyperextended position.

 (d).

Trendelenberg's test is performed with the patient standing up. The patient is asked to lift one leg off the ground. If the pelvis drops on the side of the lifted leg, there is a weakness in the abductors of the leg that the patient is standing on.

 (b).

With the patient lying on a couch, one hip is flexed up as far as it can go. A hand is passed behind the patient's back to determine whether any compensatory hyperlordosis of the lumbar spine has been eliminated by this manoeuvre. As a result, if there is any fixed flexion deformity of the other leg that is extended on the couch, it will become apparent.

(A9)   (c).

A vertical line and a horizontal line are drawn from the central point of the acetabulum, which generates the three DeLee and Charnley zones.

(A10)   (b).

Gruen zone 4 is located inferior to the tip of the prosthesis.

(A11)   (c).

The centre edge angle of Wiberg is used to determine acetabular dysplasia in patients over 5 years of age. The angle is formed by a line drawn from the centre of the femoral head to the superolateral edge of the acetabulum, and a vertical line drawn through the centre of the femoral head. An angle of > 25° is considered normal. An angle of < 20° indicates dysplasia.

(A12)   (a).

Gamma-irradiated polyethylene stored in an oxygen environment has a tendency to delaminate and crack under repetitive cyclic loading. It should therefore be stored in an inert environment. In such an environment polyethylene forms cross-links which improve wear resistance but reduce mechanical strength. Therefore cross-linked polyethylene may fail catastrophically if excess strains are applied.

(A13)   (e).

Femoral canal brushing, use of a cement gun, pulse lavage and use of a cement restrictor are techniques introduced in second-generation cementing. Although cement gun use commenced in 1971, it was formally introduced as part of the second-generation cementing technique, which began in 1975.

(A14)   (e).

Increasing the diameter of the femoral head increases the primary arc of movement, and also confers improved stability because of a more favourable head-neck ratio.

(d).

Fracture of the femoral neck has been reported in approximately 1.5% of cases after metal-on-metal hip resurfacing arthroplasty.

- Shimmin AJ, Back D. Femoral neck fractures following Birmingham hip resurfacing: a national review of 50 cases. *J Bone Joint Surg Br.* 2005; **87**: 463–4.

 (c).

The incidence of dislocation of total hip replacements is believed to be higher in patients with abnormalities of muscle tone, such as those with Parkinson's disease and those who have suffered a stroke.

- Weber M *et al.* Total hip replacement in patients with Parkinson's disease. *Int Orthop.* 2002; **26**: 66–8.

 (e).

The sciatic nerve is by far the most commonly injured nerve during total hip replacement, probably due to its proximity to the hip joint. The sciatic nerve can be injured directly by a scalpel or cutting diathermy, it can be compressed by retractors or postoperative haematoma, or cement can cause thermal injury.

- Schmalzried TP *et al.* Nerve palsy associated with total hip replacement. Risk factors and prognosis. *J Bone Joint Surg Am.* 1991; **73**: 1074–80.

(A18) (b).

Meralgia paraesthetica is a painful mononeuropathy of the lateral femoral cutaneous nerve of the thigh (LFCN). The LFCN is responsible for the sensation of the anterolateral thigh and is a purely sensory nerve. The nerve runs through the pelvis to the lateral part of the inguinal ligament. Here it passes to the thigh through a tunnel formed by the lateral attachment of the inguinal ligament and the anterior superior iliac spine. This is the commonest site of entrapment. Patients generally present with paraesthesias and numbness of the upper lateral thigh.

(A19) (b).

Acetabular protrusion is seen in a high proportion of patients who have rheumatoid arthritis.

- Gusis SE *et al*. Protrusio acetabuli in adult rheumatoid arthritis. *Clin Rheumatol*. 1991; **10**: 158–61.

(A20) (b).

All of these apart from diuretics are associated with an increased risk of avascular necrosis of the femoral head.

(A21) (a).

The psoas and iliacus muscles originate from the lumbar spine and the pelvis, respectively. The combined tendon is inserted on to the lesser trochanter of the femur. The iliopsoas is a powerful flexor of the hip and a weak external rotator. In the event of a fracture of the femoral neck, these actions are enhanced and the limb adopts a shortened and externally rotated position.

(A22) (c).

The tip–apex distance is the sum of the distance from the tip of the lag screw to the apex of the femoral head on an anteroposterior radiograph and this distance on a lateral radiograph, after controlling for magnification. If this distance is < 24 mm, fixation failure should not occur.

- Baumgaertner MR *et al*. The value of the tip–apex distance in predicting failure of fixation of peritrochanteric fractures of the hip. *J Bone Joint Surg Am*. 1995; **77**: 1058–64.

(e).

This is to allow the screw to back out as the fracture collapses. This controlled collapse is essential to allow the fragments to impact, and for the fracture to unite.

 (d).

The presence of dementia has a negative effect on functional outcome after proximal femur fractures, and such patients are less likely to return to ambulation.

- Ishida Y *et al*. Factors affecting ambulatory status and survival of patients 90 years and older with hip fractures. *Clin Orthop Relat Res*. 2005; **436**: 208–15.

 (b).

In young patients it is important to try to preserve the native femoral head. Therefore, despite the fact that there is a 30–40% failure rate associated with internal fixation of displaced intracapsular femoral neck fractures, this should be attempted.

 (d).

Screw holes below the lesser trochanter create stress risers, and consequently increase the risk of subtrochanteric fracture.

 (c).

Within 2 years of internal fixation of displaced intracapsular femoral neck fractures, a non-union rate of 33% and an avascular necrosis rate of 16% have been reported.

- Lu-Yao GL *et al*. Outcomes after displaced fractures of the femoral neck. A meta-analysis of one hundred and six published reports. *J Bone Joint Surg Am*. 1994; **76**: 15–25.

 (b).

A mean femoral neck anteversion angle of 18° in men and 14° in women has been reported. As an approximation, 15° can be considered as normal.

- Braten M *et al.* Ultrasound measurements in 50 men and 50 women. *Acta Orthop Scand.* 1992; **63**: 29–32.

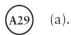 (a).

A reduced femoral head:neck ratio should raise suspicion of underlying cam-type impingement in young adults complaining of hip pain. Clinically pain is reproduced by hip flexion, adduction and internal rotation. Further evaluation with CT scanning should be performed in such cases.

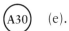 (e).

In pincer-type impingement the head:neck ratio may not be particularly reduced. However, either the acetabulum is excessively deep, or due to acetabular retroversion the femoral head or neck impinges on the acetabulum.

Section 5

Knee and lower leg

Q1 From which of the following arteries is the blood supply of the anterior cruciate ligament derived?

(a) Superior lateral geniculate artery.
(b) Superior medial geniculate artery.
(c) Middle geniculate artery.
(d) Inferior lateral geniculate artery.
(e) Inferior medial geniculate artery.

Q2 Which of the following muscles has a tendon that inserts into the pes anserinus?

(a) Semitendinosus.
(b) Semimembranosus.
(c) Biceps femoris.
(d) Adductor magnus.
(e) Popliteus.

Q3 Which of the following muscles arises from the posterior surface of the fibula, tibia and interosseous membrane?

(a) Flexor hallucis longus.
(b) Flexor digitorum longus.
(c) Extensor hallucis longus.
(d) Tibialis anterior.
(e) Tibialis posterior.

(Q4) Which of the following muscles is supplied by the superficial peroneal nerve?

(a) Tibialis anterior.
(b) Tibialis posterior.
(c) Extensor hallucis longus.
(d) Peroneus longus.
(e) Peroneus tertius.

(Q5) Which nerve supplies the muscles of the anterior compartment of the lower leg?

(a) Superficial peroneal nerve.
(b) Deep peroneal nerve.
(c) Tibal nerve.
(d) Saphenous nerve.
(e) Sural nerve.

(Q6) Which nerve supplies cutaneous innervation to the anteromedial part of the lower leg?

(a) Superficial peroneal nerve.
(b) Deep peroneal nerve.
(c) Tibal nerve.
(d) Saphenous nerve.
(e) Sural nerve.

(Q7) Which is the most sensitive test for assessing the integrity of the anterior cruciate ligament?

(a) Pivot shift test.
(b) Lachman test.
(c) Finochietto's test.
(d) Anterior drawer test.
(e) Posterior drawer test.

Q8 Which of the following examination techniques can be used to detect injuries to the posterolateral corner of the knee?

(a) Finochietto's test.
(b) Apley's grinding test.
(c) Internal rotation drawer test.
(d) External rotation drawer test.
(e) Asymmetric external rotation test.

 Q9 What is the optimal position for the knee to be in when assessing the integrity of the collateral ligaments?

(a) Full extension.
(b) Full flexion.
(c) 10° of flexion.
(d) 30° of flexion.
(e) 90° of flexion.

 Q10 A Pellegrini-Stieda lesion seen on AP radiographs of the knee is evidence of previous injury to which of the following structures?

(a) Anterior cruciate ligament.
(b) Posterior cruciate ligament.
(c) Medial collateral ligament.
(d) Patellar tendon.
(e) Medial meniscus.

 Q11 Which of the following techniques for radiographic evaluation of patellar position utilises the ratio of patellar tendon length to patella length?

(a) Insall–Salvati index.
(b) Blackburne–Peel index.
(c) Blumensaat's line.
(d) Labelle and Laurin line.
(e) Patella index.

(Q12)   What is the commonest site for an osteochondral lesion in osteochondritis dissecans of the knee?

(a)   Lateral tibal plateau.
(b)   Medial tibial plateau.
(c)   Lower pole of patella.
(d)   Anterior aspect of medial femoral condyle.
(e)   Lateral aspect of medial femoral condyle.

(Q13)   A 14-year-old girl complains of pain in her knees. The pain is exacerbated by climbing up stairs and by sitting for prolonged periods. Examination reveals a normally located patella with decreased medial translation. The girl appears to have an increased Q-angle and exhibits J-shaped patellar tracking. What is the most appropriate initial management?

(a)   Non-steroidal anti-inflammatory medication.
(b)   Four weeks of rest and activity modification.
(c)   Rehabilitation focusing on strengthening the vastus medialis obliquus.
(d)   Arthroscopic lateral release.
(e)   Tibial tubercle realignment procedure.

(Q14)   A 15-year-old boy who is a keen rugby player gives a 4-month history of pain in his left knee. On examination, tenderness is found around the distal pole of the patella. Radiographs demonstrate fragmentation of the distal pole of the patella. What is the underlying diagnosis?

(a)   Osgood–Schlatter disease.
(b)   Sinding-Larsen and Johansson syndrome.
(c)   Patellar tendinopathy.
(d)   Infrapatellar bursitis.
(e)   Osteochondritis dissecans.

Which of the following factors is a contraindication to performing a high tibial osteotomy?

(a) 10° fixed flexion deformity.
(b) 10° fixed varus deformity.
(c) Maximum flexion of 100°.
(d) Inflammatory arthritis.
(e) Medial compartment osteoarthritis.

 In which of the following conditions is patella baja most frequently seen?

(a) Previous unicompartmental knee replacement.
(b) Osgood–Schlatter disease.
(c) Sinding-Larsen and Johansson syndrome.
(d) Previous high tibial osteotomy.
(e) Previous distal femoral osteotomy.

 When performing a total knee replacement in a valgus knee, which of the following structures needs to be released if the lateral compartment is tight in flexion?

(a) Medial collateral ligament.
(b) Semimembranosus.
(c) Posterior cruciate ligament.
(d) Popliteus.
(e) Iliotibial tract.

 Which of the following is the most effective way of achieving ligament balance in the sagittal plane when performing a total knee replacement?

(a) Achieving an equal flexion and extension gap.
(b) Sacrificing the posterior cruciate ligament.
(c) Ensuring adequate medial soft tissue release.
(d) Ensuring adequate lateral soft tissue release.
(e) Ensuring that the distal femoral cut is perpendicular to the anatomical axis of the femur.

(Q19)   Which of the following advantages is associated with preservation of the posterior cruciate ligament during total knee replacement?

(a)   Decreased polyethylene wear.
(b)   Increased knee flexion.
(c)   Increased knee extension.
(d)   Improved patellar tracking.
(e)   Improved knee stability in extension.

(Q20)   Which of the following complications is specifically associated with posterior stabilised total knee replacements?

(a)   Increased polyethylene wear.
(b)   Tibial insert fracture.
(c)   Patella baja.
(d)   Patellar maltracking.
(e)   Dislocation.

(Q21)   In which of the following situations is it advantageous to use a posterior stabilised total knee replacement?

(a)   Tricompartmental osteoarthritis.
(b)   Pre-existent anterior cruciate ligament rupture.
(c)   Previous patellectomy.
(d)   Valgus deformity.
(e)   Fixed flexion deformity.

(Q22)   Which of the following technical factors does *not* help to optimise patellar tracking when performing a total knee replacement?

(a)   Neutral rotation of the tibial component.
(b)   Internal rotation of the femoral component.
(c)   Correction of valgus deformity.
(d)   Maintaining the level of the joint line.
(e)   Medial placement of the patellar component.

Which of the following factors has been implicated in the phenomenon of catastrophic wear seen after total knee replacement?

(a)   Polyethylene inserts of only 10 mm thickness.
(b)   Tibial inserts with a large contact surface area.
(c)   Tibial cuts with a posterior slope.
(d)   Posterior stabilised knee replacements.
(e)   Polyethylene gamma-sterilised in air.

 What is the most important factor governing ultimate flexion range after total knee replacement?

(a)   Soft tissue balancing.
(b)   Posterior cruciate ligament preservation.
(c)   Amount of posterior slope of tibial cut.
(d)   Preoperative range of flexion.
(e)   Postoperative use of CPM machine.

 A 36-year-old motorcyclist is seen in the emergency department after being involved in a road traffic accident. He has sustained a closed fracture to his left tibial diaphysis. Despite being given 30 mg of intramuscular morphine, he remains in pain. Examination reveals significant swelling of the lower leg, with diminished sensation anteromedially and a weak dorsalis pedis pulse. Passive movement of the toes results in severe pain. What is the underlying diagnosis?

(a)   Anterior tibial artery injury.
(b)   Saphenous nerve injury.
(c)   Compartment syndrome.
(d)   Rhabdomyolysis.
(e)   Deep vein thrombosis.

When monitoring the pressure of muscle compartments, a diagnosis of compartment syndrome can be made if the compartment pressure is which of the following?

(a)   Equal to or more than the diastolic blood pressure.
(b)   Equal to or more than the systolic blood pressure.
(c)   Equal to or more than 50% of the systolic blood pressure.
(d)   Within 30 mmHg of the diastolic blood pressure.
(e)   Within 30 mmHg of the systolic blood pressure.

 A 25-year-old footballer is involved in a poor challenge and sustains an open fracture of his right tibia. He has a wound 4 cm in diameter on the anteromedial aspect of the lower leg. The wound is heavily contaminated with mud, and extensive periosteal stripping is present. At the time of surgery the wound cannot be primarily closed due to soft tissue loss. What is the Gustilo grade of this injury?

(a)   Grade 1.
(b)   Grade 2.
(c)   Grade 3a.
(d)   Grade 3b.
(e)   Grade 3c.

 A 23-year-old woman is reviewed in the outpatient clinic 8 months after undergoing intramedullary nailing for a tibial shaft fracture. Her fracture had been slow to unite, and after 2 months the intramedullary nail was dynamised. Current radiographs still confirm a hypertrophic non-union. What is the most appropriate course of management?

(a)   Exchange nailing with a larger nail.
(b)   Immobilisation in a plaster cast.
(c)   Internal fixation with a locking plate.
(d)   Nail removal and Ilizarov frame application.
(e)   Pulsed low-intensity ultrasound treatment.

According to the Schatzker classification, what grade is a split depression of the lateral tibial plateau?

(a) Grade I.
(b) Grade II.
(c) Grade III.
(d) Grade IV.
(e) Grade V.

 What is the potential complication associated with arthroscopy in the management of tibial plateau fractures?

(a) Fat embolism.
(b) Deep vein thrombosis.
(c) Infection.
(d) Popliteal artery injury.
(e) Compartment syndrome.

 What is the incidence of arterial injury in dislocation of the knee?

(a) 1%.
(b) 10%.
(c) 20%.
(d) 33%.
(e) 50%.

 With regard to dislocation of the knee, which of the following statements is true?

(a) Knee dislocation only occurs with rupture of both cruciate ligaments.
(b) The tibial nerve is the most commonly injured nerve.
(c) Spontaneous reduction occurs in a significant number of cases.
(d) Successful closed reduction should be followed by urgent arthroscopic evaluation.
(e) When both cruciate ligaments are ruptured, the anterior cruciate ligament should be repaired first.

Q33 With regard to the evaluation of arterial injury after knee dislocation, which of the following statements is true?

(a)   Routine arteriography should always be performed.
(b)   The presence of pedal pulses excludes an underlying arterial injury.
(c)   If pedal pulses remain absent after reduction of the knee, an MR arteriogram should be obtained.
(d)   Arteriography is more likely to be required in anterior knee dislocations.
(e)   If physical examination reveals no evidence of arterial injury, arteriography is not required.

 Q34 A 45-year-old front-seat passenger is involved in a road traffic accident. He banged his knee against the dashboard and sustained a minimally displaced transverse fracture of the patella. Which of the following factors is most important in determining management of this injury?

(a)   The ability to extend the knee.
(b)   The amount of fracture displacement.
(c)   The degree of knee swelling.
(d)   The amount of pain.
(e)   The ability to weight bear.

 Q35 A 67-year-old woman is brought to the emergency department with a 12-hour history of left knee pain. She is generally fit and well and takes no regular medication. She gives no history of injury, but has been feeling cold and shivery. Her temperature is 39.2°C, and the knee is swollen, erythematous and warm. She is holding her knee in 20° of flexion and is unwilling to allow any movement. Her blood parameters reveal a WBC of 16.9×10^9/l, an ESR of 78 mm/ hour, a CRP of 157 mg/L and a raised serum uric acid concentration. What is the most appropriate form of treatment?

(a)   Intravenous antibiotics.
(b)   Non-steroidal anti-inflammatory drugs.

(c)   Allopurinol.
(d)   Knee joint aspiration.
(e)   Arthroscopic washout of the knee joint.

Answers

 (c).

The middle geniculate artery arises approximately at the level of the joint line and passes anteriorly to pierce the oblique popliteal ligament and posterior joint capsule. It traverses the posterior joint capsule at the level of the intercondylar notch and supplies the anterior and posterior cruciate ligaments.

 (a).

The semitendinosus originates at the ischial tuberosity, along with the tendon of the biceps femoris, and inserts into the pes anserinus. The semitendinosus flexes and medially rotates the calf at the knee.

 (e).

The tibialis posterior originates from the lateral part of the posterior surface of the tibia, the medial two-thirds of the fibula, the interosseous membrane, intermuscular septum and deep fascia. It runs in the posterior compartment of the lower leg, passing behind the medial malleolus, before the major part inserts into the navicular tuberosity. Smaller slips also pass to the sustentaculum tali, the plantar surface of all three cuneiforms, the cuboid and the bases of the second, third and fourth metatarsal bones. Its primary action is to invert and plantarflex the foot at the ankle.

 (d).

The peroneus longus originates from the lateral condyle of the tibia, the head and proximal two-thirds of the lateral surface of the fibula, the intermuscular septum and adjacent fascia. It typically runs posterior to the tendon of the peroneus brevis, and passes inferior to the cuboid before inserting into the lateral margin of the plantar surface of the first cuneiform and the proximal end of the first metatarsal.

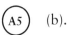 (b).

The deep peroneal nerve is a branch of the common peroneal nerve. The common peroneal nerve courses anteriorly around the neck of the fibula, and lies on the anterior cortex of the fibula, beneath the peroneus longus muscle. Here it divides into its deep and superficial branches. The deep peroneal nerve is accompanied by the anterior tibial artery, as it passes distally lying between the tibialis anterior and the extensor hallucis longus. It supplies all of the muscles of the anterior compartment of the lower leg, and gives a sensory branch to the first web space of the foot.

 (d).

The saphenous nerve arises from the femoral nerve in the femoral triangle. It passes down in the femoral triangle to enter the adductor canal. It then pierces the fascia lata between the tendons of the sartorius and gracilis, and passes inferiorly on the medial side of the leg close to the greater saphenous vein.

 (b).

The Lachman test is most sensitive for determining ruptures of the anterior cruciate ligament. The pivot shift test is highly specific but lacks sensitivity.

- Prins M. The Lachman test is the most sensitive and the pivot shift the most specific test for the diagnosis of ACL rupture. *Aust J Physiother.* 2006; **52:** 66.
- Solomon DH *et al.* The rational clinical examination. Does this patient have a torn meniscus or ligament of the knee? Value of the physical examination. *JAMA.* 2001; **286:** 1610–20.

 (e).

The patient lies in a prone position, and the feet are externally rotated in 30° and 90° of knee flexion. Increased external rotation of more than 10–15° indicates a posterolateral corner injury.

Increased external rotation at both 30° and 90° of knee flexion indicates a posterolateral corner injury along with a posterior cruciate ligament rupture.

 (d).

In full extension, the posterior cruciate ligament and the articulation of the femoral condyles with the proximal tibia stabilise the knee. With increasing knee flexion, the strong anteromedial component of the anterior cruciate ligament stabilises the knee. Consequently, 30° of knee flexion is the optimal position for determining the integrity of the collateral ligaments.

 (c).

A Pellegrini-Stieda lesion occurs secondary to an avulsion of the medial collateral ligament from the medial femoral condyle. Over time, calcification occurs in the superior portion of the medial collateral ligament. Therefore the presence of a Pellegrini-Stieda lesion on radiographs is a chronic sign representing a previous injury to the medial collateral ligament.

 (a).

The Blackburne–Peel index compares the ratio of the patellar articular surface length to the distance of the tibial plateau from the inferior part of the patellar articular surface. With 30° of knee flexion, Blumensaat's line should pass from the inferior border of the patella through the intercondylar notch. With the knee flexed to 90°, the patella should lie between a line drawn along the anterior and posterior femoral cortices. The patellar index assesses patellar alignment.

 (e).

Although osteochondritis dissecans can occur in any part of the knee, the commonest location is the lateral aspect of the medial femoral condyle.

(A13) (c).

The young girl in this clinical scenario is suffering from anterior knee pain. The first line of management is rehabilitation, focusing on strengthening the vastus medialis obliquus muscle. This helps to keep the patella medialised, thus preventing excessive wear on the lateral patellar articular facet. If after 6 to 12 months of rehabilitation there has been no improvement, surgery can be considered.

(A14) (b).

Sinding-Larsen and Johansson syndrome is characterised by pain and tenderness over the inferior pole of the patella. Symptoms of infrapatellar pain and limping are precipitated by overstraining or trauma. A slightly swollen, warm and tender bump just below the kneecap, and pain during activity or following an extended period of vigorous exercise in adolescents is typical of this condition.

(A15) (d).

A high tibial osteotomy can be performed in patients under 60 years of age with medial compartment arthritis, less than 15° of fixed flexion deformity, 10–12° of varus deformity, and active flexion to 90°. More than 20° of required correction, lateral joint space narrowing and inflammatory arthritis are contraindications to this procedure.

- Dennis MG, Di Cesare PE. Surgical management of the middle-age arthritic knee. *Bull Hosp Jt Dis.* 2003; **61:** 172–8.

(A16) (d).

- Kesmezacar H *et al.* Evaluation of patellar height and measurement methods after valgus high tibial osteotomy. *Knee Surg Sports Traumatol Arthrosc.* 2005; **13:** 539–44.

(A17) (d).

The iliotibial band should be released if the knee is tight in extension. The medial collateral ligament, semimembranosus, and posterior cruciate ligament should be released for varus deformities.

(a).

Once an equal extension and flexion gap is achieved, the ligaments should become balanced.

 (b).

Preserving the posterior cruciate ligament facilitates femoral rollback, which allows greater flexion to be achieved. However, this has the disadvantage of increasing polyethylene wear. Posterior cruciate ligament preservation improves stability in flexion, not in extension.

 (e).

As mentioned previously, posterior cruciate ligament preservation increases polyethylene wear. Therefore sacrificing the posterior cruciate ligament actually reduces polyethylene wear. With posterior stabilised knee replacements, the femoral component can jump over the tibial post. In such a situation, manipulation under anaesthesia is required to achieve reduction.

 (c).

Patellectomy reduces the strength of the quadriceps by up to 30%. Anterior femoral displacement tends to occur as a result of the decreased quadriceps strength. This reduces the amount of effective flexion that can be achieved. Therefore it is advantageous to use a posterior stabilised knee which prevents anterior femoral displacement.

 (b).

The femoral component should be positioned in 3° of external rotation. This ensures that the distal femoral cut is parallel to the tibia, which helps to achieve an equal extension and flexion gap. This is turn ensures that the soft tissues are balanced, which helps to maintain patellar tracking.

(A23) (e).

Oxidised polyethylene has dimished mechanical properties, which render it susceptible to delamination and subsurface cracking. This can result in catastrophic wear and early failure of implants. Provided that the polyethylene thickness is greater than 8 mm, the risk of catastrophic wear should not be increased.

(A24) (d).

The amount of flexion achieved after total knee replacement is most significantly determined by the preoperative range of flexion. Usually flexion within $10°$ of the preoperative amount is achieved, assuming that technically accurate surgery has been performed. Technical deficiencies can result in a significantly reduced range of motion.

(A25) (c).

Compartment syndrome is a potentially serious complication associated with tibial fractures. It is more common with closed injuries occurring in young males. However, it can occur with open injuries. Pain that is out of proportion to the injury should raise suspicion of this complication. Classically, severe pain occurs on passive movement of the toes. If the diagnosis is uncertain, compartment pressure monitoring may be performed.

(A26) (d).

However, it should be noted that even with lower pressures, if clinical suspicion is high, it may be prudent to perform a fasciotomy.

(A27) (d).

Despite the fact that the diameter of the wound is less than 10 cm, this becomes a grade 3 injury in view of the extensive contamination and periosteal stripping. As soft tissue has been lost and cover cannot be achieved, it becomes a grade 3b injury.

(a).

A hypertrophic non-union tends to indicate that fracture union has not occurred because of mechanical instability. Dynamisation of the nail at 2 months can be viewed as inappropriate, as tibial fractures often take up to 4 months to unite. Although any method of improving fracture stability can be employed, exchange nailing results in better outcomes, as reaming of the canal appears to stimulate fracture union.

 (b).

Grade I is a lateral condyle split, Grade II is a split depression of the lateral condyle, Grade III is a pure depression, Grade IV is a fracture of the medial condyle, Grade V is a bicondylar fracture and Grade VI is a uni/bicondylar fracture with complete meta-diaphyseal dissociation.

 (e).

Compartment syndrome can occur as a result of fluid extravasation into the soft tissues of the lower leg.

- Belanger M, Fadale P. Compartment syndrome of the leg after arthroscopic examination of a tibial plateau fracture. Case report and review of the literature. *Arthroscopy*. 1997; **13**: 646–51.

 (d).

 (c).

Knee dislocation can occur with rupture of only one cruciate ligament. The common peroneal nerve is the most commonly injured nerve. Acute arthroscopic evaluation is relatively contraindicated, as capsular injury predisposes to development of compartment syndrome. The posterior cruciate ligament is the cornerstone of the knee, and should be repaired first. Tightening the anterior cruciate in the presence of a posterior cruciate rupture results in posterior subluxation of the tibia. Many knee dislocations can reduce spontaneously. Therefore in cases of significant trauma it is essential to maintain a high index of suspicion.

(e).

Even if pedal pulses are palpable, an underlying intimal injury may be present. If pedal pulses do not return after reduction of the knee, time should not be wasted in obtaining an arteriogram, and the patient should be taken to theatre urgently for surgical exploration. Posterior knee dislocations have a higher incidence of arterial injury. If serial physical examinations are satisfactory, arteriography is not routinely required in knee dislocations.

- Hollis JD, Daley BJ. 10-year review of knee dislocations: is arteriography always necessary? *J Trauma*. 2005; **59**: 672–6.
- Stannard JP *et al*. Vascular injuries in knee dislocations: the role of physical examination in determining the need for arteriography. *J Bone Joint Surg Am*. 2004; **86-A**: 910–15.

(A34) (a).

Provided that the patient can straight leg raise actively, a minimally displaced transverse fracture of the patella can be managed non-operatively. However, if straight leg raising cannot be achieved, surgical fixation is required.

(A35) (d).

This woman may be suffering from septic arthritis. However, given the raised uric acid level, she may also be suffering from gout. Arthrocentesis, and analysis of the aspirate for organisms and crystals, is the appropriate first-line management. If the diagnosis is septic arthritis, washout of the knee joint is indicated. However, if the diagnosis is gout, symptomatic treatment with non-steroidal anti-inflammatory drugs is indicated.

Section 6

Foot and ankle

Q1 Which of the following nerves supplies sensory innervation to the first web space of the foot?

(a) Superficial peroneal nerve.
(b) Deep peroneal nerve.
(c) Sural nerve.
(d) Saphenous nerve.
(e) Tibial nerve.

Q2 Which of the following nerves is at risk in the lateral approach to the distal fibula?

(a) Superficial peroneal nerve.
(b) Deep peroneal nerve.
(c) Sural nerve.
(d) Saphenous nerve.
(e) Tibial nerve.

Q3 Of which nerve is the medial dorsal cutaneous nerve of the foot, which is at risk during surgery to the first metatarsophalangeal joint, a terminal branch?

(a) Superficial peroneal nerve.
(b) Deep peroneal nerve.
(c) Sural nerve.
(d) Saphenous nerve.
(e) Tibial nerve.

Q4 Which of the following muscles is the primary plantar-flexor of the first metatarsal?

(a) Tibialis posterior.
(b) Flexor hallucis longus.
(c) Flexor digitorum longus.
(d) Peroneus brevis.
(e) Peroneus longus.

Q5 On the medial side of the ankle, which of the following structures is located most posteriorly?

(a) Tibialis posterior.
(b) Flexor digitorum longus.
(c) Flexor hallucis longus.
(d) Posterior tibial artery.
(e) Tibial nerve.

Q6 On the dorsum of the foot, what is the position of the dorsalis pedis artery?

(a) Medial to the tibialis anterior.
(b) Medial to the extensor hallucis longus.
(c) Lateral to the extensor digitorum longus.
(d) Between the extensor hallucis longus and the extensor digitorum longus.
(e) Between the tibialis anterior and the extensor hallucis longus.

Q7 Which of the following bones are connected by the spring ligament?

(a) Talus and navicular.
(b) Calcaneus and navicular.
(c) Calcaneus and talus.
(d) Calcaneus and cuboid.
(e) Talus and fibula.

Q8 Which of the following ligaments is tested when an anterior drawer test is performed on the ankle with the foot in a plantar-flexed position?

(a) Anterior talofibular ligament.
(b) Posterior talofibular ligament.
(c) Calcaneofibular ligament.
(d) Anterior tibiofibular ligament.
(e) Deltoid ligament.

Q9 The tendon of which of the following muscles grooves both the talus and the sustentaculum tali as it passes into the foot?

(a) Tibialis posterior.
(b) Flexor digitorum longus.
(c) Flexor hallucis longus.
(d) Peroneus longus.
(e) Peroneus brevis.

Q10 In the tendon of which muscle are the medial and lateral sesamoids associated with the first metatarsal head located?

(a) Flexor digitorum longus.
(b) Flexor hallucis longus.
(c) Flexor hallucis brevis.
(d) Abductor hallucis.
(e) Adductor hallucis.

Q11 What is the upper limit of normal for the intermetatarsal angle between the first and second ray?

(a) 4°.
(b) 9°.
(c) 15°.
(d) 20°.
(e) 25°.

(Q12) What is the upper limit of normal for the hallux valgus angle?

(a) 4°.
(b) 9°.
(c) 15°.
(d) 20°.
(e) 25°.

(Q13) A 55-year-old woman complains of pain in her left foot between the third and fourth metatarsal heads. The pain is burning in nature and is exacerbated by weight bearing. Compression between the third and fourth metatarsal heads reproduces her pain, and she also has altered sensation of the third and fourth toes. What is the underlying diagnosis?

(a) Morton's neuroma.
(b) Metatarsal stress fracture.
(c) Metatarsophalangeal joint synovitis.
(d) Freiberg's infraction.
(e) Plantar keratosis.

(Q14) What is the success rate after excision of a Morton's neuroma?

(a) 10%.
(b) 30%.
(c) 50%.
(d) 80%.
(e) 95%.

(Q15) A 36-year-old man complains of pain and numbness on the medial side of his right foot and ankle. The pain is reproduced by tapping behind the medial malleolus. What is the likely underlying diagnosis?

(a) Plantar fasciitis.
(b) Tibialis posterior tendon dysfunction.

(c)   Talonavicular joint arthritis.
(d)   Deltoid ligament rupture.
(e)   Tarsal tunnel syndrome.

 Q16   A 15-year-old boy is seen in the outpatient clinic. He gives a 6-month history of difficulty in walking, with recurrent falls and ankle sprains. He is noted to have wasting of the calf muscles and walks with a high-stepping gait. His feet have high medial longitudinal arches, and hindfoot varus is present. He has absent ankle jerks and diminished proprioception of his toes. What is the underlying diagnosis?

(a)   Diabetic peripheral neuropathy.
(b)   Charcot–Marie–Tooth disease.
(c)   Leprosy.
(d)   Juvenile rheumatoid arthritis.
(e)   Cerebral palsy.

 Q17   In a pes cavus deformity, relative weakness of which of the following muscles is observed?

(a)   Extensor hallucis longus.
(b)   Extensor digitorum longus.
(c)   Tibialis anterior.
(d)   Tibialis posterior.
(e)   Peroneus longus.

 Q18   Which of the following is *not* a recognised feature of pes cavus deformity?

(a)   Hindfoot varus.
(b)   First ray plantar flexion.
(c)   Forefoot adduction.
(d)   Forefoot supination.
(e)   Great toe cock-up deformity.

(Q19) In the evaluation of pes cavus, which of the following does the Coleman block help to determine?

(a)   Flexibility of hindfoot varus.
(b)   Flexibility of the forefoot.
(c)   Intrinsic muscle weakness.
(d)   The medial longitudinal arch.
(e)   The ankle joint.

(Q20) In which of the following conditions do patients characteristically complain that pain is most severe with the first few steps in the morning?

(a)   Interdigital neuroma.
(b)   Lateral plantar nerve compression.
(c)   Freiberg's infraction.
(d)   Plantar fasciitis.
(e)   Achilles tendinopathy.

(Q21) What is the most appropriate first line of treatment in plantar fasciitis?

(a)   Steroid injection.
(b)   Night splintage.
(c)   Physiotherapy.
(d)   Surgical release of the plantar fascia.
(e)   Complete resection of the plantar fascia.

(Q22) Which of the following complications is characteristically associated with steroid injections into the plantar fascia?

(a)   Flexor digitorum brevis rupture.
(b)   Lateral plantar nerve injury.
(c)   Medial calcaneal nerve injury.
(d)   Calcaneal osteomyelitis.
(e)   Fat pad atrophy.

A 45-year-old man gives a 4-week history of pain in his heel. The pain has developed insidiously and he gives no history of trauma. He has a sedentary job, but in the last 2 months has started jogging in order to try to lose weight. Clinically he is tender over the proximal plantar fascia and also complains of pain on compression of the calcaneus. Plain radiographs do not show any abnormality. Which of the following would be the investigation of choice to aid diagnosis?

(a)   MRI scan.
(b)   Bone scan.
(c)   CT scan.
(d)   Ultrasound scan.
(e)   Nerve conduction studies.

 A 45-year-old woman complains of pain on the medial side of her ankle. On examination she displays the 'too many toes' sign, and is unable to perform a single leg heel raise. What is the most likely diagnosis?

(a)   Tarsal tunnel syndrome.
(b)   Flexor hallucis longus rupture.
(c)   Tarsal coalition.
(d)   Deltoid ligament strain.
(e)   Tibialis posterior tendon dysfunction.

 Which of the following is the principal antagonist of the tibialis posterior muscle?

(a)   Peroneus brevis.
(b)   Peroneus longus.
(c)   Tibialis anterior.
(d)   Extensor digitorum longus.
(e)   Flexor digitorum brevis.

Which of the following is not observed in tibialis posterior tendon dysfunction?

(a) Loss of the medial longitudinal arch.
(b) Forefoot abduction.
(c) Forefoot pronation.
(d) Hindfoot valgus.
(e) Hindfoot equinus.

 A 51-year-old woman with tibialis posterior tendon dysfunction complains of pain in the lateral aspect of her ankle. On examination she is unable to perform a single heel raise on the affected limb. She has fixed hindfoot valgus, and the flatfoot deformity cannot be corrected. Subtalar joint movements are stiff and lead to discomfort, but ankle movements are complete and pain free. What stage of tibialis posterior tendon dysfunction is she suffering from?

(a) I.
(b) II.
(c) III.
(d) IV.
(e) V.

 A 47-year-old man complains of pain on the medial side of his ankle. On examination he displays the 'too many toes' sign. His hindfoot is in valgus, and he is unable to perform a single heel raise on the affected side. His hindfoot valgus and flatfoot deformity are fixed. He has limited, painful movement of the subtalar joint, although ankle joint movement is complete and pain free. What would be the most appropriate form of management for this patient?

(a) Ankle foot orthosis.
(b) Debridement of the tibialis posterior tendon.
(c) Calcaneal osteotomy.
(d) Flexor digitorum longus to tibialis posterior tendon transfer.
(e) Triple arthrodesis.

Q29 What is the main advantage of surgical repair of Achilles tendon ruptures compared with non-operative management?

(a) Improved tendon excursion.
(b) Decreased re-rupture rate.
(c) Improved tensile strength.
(d) Decreased inpatient stay.
(e) Decreased complication rate.

 Q30 Use of which of the following groups of antibiotics has been associated with an increased incidence of Achilles tendinopathy?

(a) Penicillins.
(b) Cephalosporins.
(c) Aminoglycosides.
(d) Fluoroquinolones.
(e) Macrolides.

 Q31 What is the most common location of osteochondral lesions of the talus?

(a) Anteromedial.
(b) Anterolateral.
(c) Central.
(d) Posteromedial.
(e) Posterolateral.

 Q32 A 24-year-old ballet dancer complains of pain in her ankle. Clinically, she is tender posterior to the peroneal tendons and her pain is reproduced with forced plantar flexion of the ankle. What is the most likely underlying diagnosis?

(a) Peroneal tendon subluxation.
(b) Sinus tarsi syndrome.
(c) Tarsal coalition.
(d) Fibular avulsion fracture.
(e) Os trigonum syndrome.

Q33 In equinus deformity of the ankle, which of the following tests is used to assess gastrocnemius tightness?

(a) Simmond's test.
(b) Thompson's test.
(c) Silfverskiold test.
(d) Coleman block test.
(e) Cotton test.

Q34 An 18-year-old man complains of recurrent left ankle sprains and discomfort when walking on uneven surfaces. On examination he has a reduced left medial arch. He is tender over the lateral aspect of the left foot, and has reduced subtalar joint motion. What is the most likely underlying diagnosis?

(a) Peroneal tendon subluxation.
(b) Sinus tarsi syndrome.
(c) Os trigonum syndrome.
(d) Tarsal coalition.
(e) Tibialis posterior tendon dysfunction.

Q35 What is the most significant risk associated with isolated fractures of the medial malleolus?

(a) Avascular necrosis.
(b) Non-union.
(c) Saphenous nerve injury.
(d) Tibialis posterior tendon injury.
(e) Ankle impingement.

Q36 Which of the following is not a component of the ankle syndesmosis?

(a) Deltoid ligament.
(b) Anterior inferior tibiofibular ligament.
(c) Posterior inferior tibiofibular ligament.
(d) Inferior transverse ligament.
(e) Interosseous membrane.

(Q37) To which type of Lauge-Hansen injury is a Weber C fibular fracture equivalent?

(a)   Supination – external rotation.
(b)   Supination – adduction.
(c)   Supination – abduction.
(d)   Pronation – abduction.
(e)   Pronation – external rotation.

(Q38) What is the most significant complication of talar neck fractures?

(a)   Avascular necrosis.
(b)   Non-union.
(c)   Dorsalis pedis injury.
(d)   Flexor hallucis longus injury.
(e)   Ankle impingement.

(Q39) A 43-year-old man who was involved in a road traffic accident sustained a fracture of his talus. Radiographs show a fracture through the talar neck with dislocation of both ankle and subtalar joints. What grade of Hawkins classification does this correspond to?

(a)   I.
(b)   II.
(c)   III.
(d)   IV.
(e)   V.

(Q40) In the above case, what is the incidence of avascular necrosis likely to be?

(a)   10%.
(b)   25%.
(c)   50%.
(d)   75%.
(e)   100%.

(Q41) In patients who have sustained a fracture of the calcaneum, there is a high incidence of also having sustained a fracture of which other bone?

(a) Cuboid.
(b) Metatarsals.
(c) Tibial plateau.
(d) Lumbar vertebra.
(e) Femoral neck.

(Q42) What is the normal value of Bohler's angle?

(a) 5–10°.
(b) 10–20°.
(c) 20–40°.
(d) 40–60°.
(e) 60–80°.

(Q43) Which nerve is at risk during open reduction and internal fixation of calcaneal fractures?

(a) Saphenous nerve.
(b) Sural nerve.
(c) Deep peroneal nerve.
(d) Superficial peroneal nerve.
(e) Tibial nerve.

(Q44) In the midfoot, the Lisfranc ligament connects which of the following bones?

(a) Medial cuneiform to second metatarsal.
(b) Medial cuneiform to first metatarsal.
(c) Middle cuneiform to second metatarsal.
(d) Middle cuneiform to first metatarsal.
(e) Lateral cuneiform to second metatarsal.

When performing an open reduction and internal fixation for a Lisfranc fracture dislocation, reduction of which of the metatarsal bases is the key to reduction and stability?

(a)   First.
(b)   Second.
(c)   Third.
(d)   Fourth.
(e)   Fifth.

Answers

   (b).

The deep peroneal nerve is a branch of the common peroneal nerve. The common peroneal nerve courses anteriorly around the neck of the fibula, and lies on the anterior cortex of the fibula, beneath the peroneus longus muscle. Here it divides into its deep and superficial branches. The deep peroneal nerve is accompanied by the anterior tibial artery, as it passes distally lying between the tibialis anterior and extensor hallucis longus. It supplies all of the muscles of the anterior compartment of the lower leg, and gives a sensory branch to the first web space of the foot.

   (a).

The superficial peroneal nerve supplies the peronei longus and brevis and the skin over the greater part of the dorsum of the foot. It passes forward between the peronei and the extensor digitorum longus, it pierces the deep fascia at the lower third of the leg, and is vulnerable to injury here in the approach to the lateral malleolus.

   (a).

The medial dorsal cutaneous nerve of the foot is a branch of the superficial peroneal nerve. It passes in front of the ankle joint, and divides into two dorsal digital branches, one of which supplies the medial side of the great toe, while the other supplies the adjacent side of the second and third toes.

 (e).

The peroneus longus originates from the lateral condyle of the tibia, the head and proximal two-thirds of the lateral surface of the fibula, the intermuscular septum and adjacent fascia. It typically runs posterior to the tendon of the peroneus brevis, and passes inferior to the cuboid before inserting into the lateral margin of the plantar surface of the first cuneiform and the proximal end of the first metatarsal.

 (c).

The structures on the medial side of the ankle are arranged in the following order: Tibialis posterior, flexor Digitorum longus, Artery, Nerve, flexor Hallucis longus (mnemonic – Tall Doctors Are Never Happy.)

 (d).

The dorsalis pedis artery is the continuation of the anterior tibial artery. It passes forward from the ankle joint along the tibial side of the dorsum of the foot to the proximal part of the first inter-metatarsal space, where it divides into two branches, the first dorsal metatarsal and the deep plantar. On its medial side is the tendon of the extensor hallucis longus. On its lateral side are the first tendon of the extensor digitorum longus, and the termination of the deep peroneal nerve.

 (b).

The spring ligament is composed of the inferior calcaneonavicular and superomedial calcaneonavicular ligaments and a third component which runs from the notch between the anterior and middle calcaneal facets to the tubercle of the navicular. It plays a role in supporting the head of the talus.

(a).

The anterior talofibular ligament (ATFL) is a thickening of the ankle capsule. It passes from the anterior margin of the lateral malleolus, forward and medially, to the talus, in front of its lateral articular facet. The ATFL is the weakest of the lateral ligaments. Strain in the ATFL is minimal in dorsiflexion and neutral, and increases as the ankle progressively moves into plantar flexion.

 (c).

The flexor hallucis longus originates from the distal two-thirds of the posterior fibula, interosseous membrane and adjacent inter-muscular septum. It passes behind the medial malleolus, and grooves both the talus and the sustentaculum tali as it passes into the plantar aspect of the foot. At the knot of Henry the tendon passes superior to the tendon of the flexor digitorum longus, crossing it from lateral to medial. It runs forward between the two heads of the flexor hallucis brevis, and is inserted into the base of the distal phalanx of the great toe. The flexor hallucis longus flexes the great toe at the foot and assists in plantar flexion of the foot at the ankle.

 (c).

The flexor hallucis brevis originates from the medial portion of the plantar surface of the cuboid bone and the adjacent portion of the lateral cuneiform bone. The medial and lateral heads of the flexor hallucis brevis insert on to the medial and lateral sesamoid bones at the first metatarsophalangeal joint, which are attached to the medial and lateral sides of the proximal phalanx of the great toe. The flexor hallucis brevis flexes the first metatarsophalangeal joint.

 (b).

From 9–15° is graded as a mild deformity, from 15–20° is graded as a moderate deformity, and greater than 20° is graded as a severe deformity.

 (c).

(A13)   (a).

Morton's neuroma usually occurs in the second or third web space. It is rare in the first or fourth web spaces. It is believed to occur secondary to repetitive trauma or traction. Typical physical findings include tenderness in the area, differential sensory loss in the affected toes, and reproduction of pain on compression of the metatarsal heads.

(A14)   (d).

80% of patients improve with surgery, although a recurrent neuroma can form 1–4 years after surgery. Patient education and footwear modification can also be successful. High success rates have also been reported with steroid injection, but this may be associated with a high incidence of late relapse.

(A15)   (e).

Tarsal tunnel syndrome occurs as a result of compression of the posterior tibial nerve, behind the medial malleolus. Compression can result from a tendon sheath ganglion, a lipoma, venous engorgement, an exostosis or fracture fragment, or neurilemoma. MRI helps to confirm and localize anatomical abnormalities. Although nerve conduction studies are often unhelpful, when positive they do confirm the diagnosis.

(A16)   (b).

Charcot–Marie–Tooth disease, also known as hereditary motor sensory neuropathy, is a disorder characterised by peroneal muscle weakness. The condition results in a pes cavus deformity. The peroneus longus overpowers the tibialis anterior, resulting in a dropped first ray. The tibialis posterior overpowers the peroneus brevis, and hindfoot varus and forefoot adduction occur as a result. Intrinsic muscle imbalance causes clawing of the toes. Muscular weakness can result in ankle instability, accounting for recurrent falls and sprains.

(A17)   (c).

The tibialis anterior and peroneus brevis are relatively weaker than the tibialis posterior and peroneus longus, respectively. To compensate for a weak tibialis anterior, the long toe extensors are recruited to help ankle dorsiflexion. This may result in cock-up deformities of the toes.

 (d).

Forefoot pronation is seen as opposed to forefoot supination. See previous text for an explanation of the other deformities seen in pes cavus.

 (a).

The Coleman block test is performed by having the patient stand with a one-inch wooden block under the heel and lateral foot. This allows the first ray to be plantar flexed off the block. If the hindfoot corrects to a neutral position, the deformity is flexible. If the hindfoot does not correct, the deformity is rigid. The test evaluates the subtalar joint and determines whether hindfoot varus is correctable or fixed. This helps to determine management. If hindfoot varus is correctable, a soft tissue procedure can help to correct the deformity, but if it is fixed, a bony procedure will be required.

 (d).

During sleep, the foot adopts an equinus position, and the plantar fascia relaxes. When taking the first few steps in the morning, the plantar fascia is stretched and microtears may also occur. As a result, intense pain is felt.

 (c).

Plantar fasciitis is a degenerative condition of the plantar fascia, rather than an inflammatory condition. Physiotherapy to stretch the plantar fascia, and patient education along with footwear modification are appropriate first-line management for this condition. Around 80% of cases resolve spontaneously within 12 months. Only 5% of patients require surgical release when non-operative measures fail.

(A22) (e).

Although all of the above complications are possible, and have been reported, fat pad atrophy and rupture of the plantar fascia are the two complications characteristically associated with steroid injection.

(A23) (b).

The two main differential diagnoses in this clinical scenario are plantar fasciitis and a stress fracture of the calcaneum. A radio-isotope bone scan is appropriate to investigate both of these conditions. It will show increased uptake around the fracture line, or increased uptake around the medial tubercle of the calcaneum and overlying periosteum.

(A24) (e).

Tibialis posterior tendon dysfunction is a condition characterised by medial ankle pain, weakness of single leg raising, and the 'too many toes' sign. A progressive pes planus deformity develops.

(A25) (a).

The primary antagonist of the posterior tibial tendon is the peroneus brevis muscle, which everts the hindfoot and abducts the midfoot.

- Pomeroy GC *et al.* Acquired flatfoot in adults due to dysfunction of the posterior tibial tendon. *J Bone Joint Surg Am.* 1999; **81:** 1173–82.

(A26) (c).

Forefoot supination rather than pronation is seen once hindfoot valgus is corrected. It is important to determine whether the forefoot supination is correctable or fixed. If the supination is fixed, additional bony correction of the midfoot may be required to correct the foot deformity.

(A27) (c).

In tibialis posterior tendon dysfunction, a fixed deformity with degenerative changes of the subtalar joint is classified as stage III. Stage IV occurs when degenerative changes affect the ankle joint.

- Johnson KA, Strom DE. Tibialis posterior tendon dysfunction. *Clin Orthop Relat Res.* 1989; **239**: 196–206.

 (e).

This clinical scenario describes stage III tibialis posterior tendon dysfunction. Therefore only triple arthrodesis is an appropriate form of management. The other treatment options can be employed in the earlier stages of tibialis posterior tendon dysfunction.

 (b).

Although a higher tensile strength is achieved with surgery, the difference is small, at around 10%. Open operative treatment of acute Achilles tendon ruptures significantly reduces the risk of re-rupture compared with non-operative treatment. Therefore the main benefit of surgical treatment is a reduced re-rupture rate.

- Khan RJK *et al.* Treatment of acute Achilles tendon ruptures. A meta-analysis of randomised, controlled trials. *J Bone Joint Surg Am.* 2005; **87**: 2202–10.

 (d).

There are numerous reports of Achilles tendon rupture associated with fluoroquinolone use.

- Sharma P, Maffulli N. Tendon injury and tendinopathy: healing and repair. *J Bone Joint Surg Am.* 2005; **87**: 187–202.

(A31) (d).

The mechanism of these injuries is inversion when the ankle is in a plantar-flexed position.

A32 (e).

Os trigonum syndrome is common in ballet dancers and results in posterior ankle impingement.

A33 (c).

Simmond's test and Thompson's test are different names for the same test, which assesses the integrity of the Achilles tendon. The Coleman block test is used to assess hindfoot varus correction in pes cavus, and the cotton test is used to assess ankle syndesmosis integrity. The Silfverskiold test assesses gastrocnemius tightness. If more ankle motion occurs with the knee flexed, this indicates that tightness is mainly due to a proximal gastrocnemius lesion, so proximal release is required. If flexion does not change ankle motion, tendon lengthening is required.

A34 (d).

Tarsal coalition is the abnormal union of two or more bones in the hindfoot and midfoot. This union may be either complete or incomplete, and the condition may be either congenital or acquired secondary to trauma, infection, surgery or articular disorders. The two commonest types, calcaneonavicular and talocalcaneal, represent the majority of tarsal coalitions.

A35 (b).

Non-union is the most significant risk. There is a 5–15% non-union rate with fractures that are displaced more than 2 mm. Therefore all displaced fractures should be fixed.

A36 (a).

The ankle syndesmosis stabilises the distal tibia and fibula. Structures connecting the distal tibia and fibula are components of the ankle syndesmosis. The deltoid ligament connects the medial malleolus to the navicular and the talus, and is therefore not a component of the ankle syndesmosis.

A37 (e).

A Weber C fracture is a fracture of the distal fibula above the level of the ankle syndesmosis. The Lauge-Hansen classification is based on the mechanism of injury. Pronation and external rotation will result in a fracture of the distal fibula above the level of the syndesmosis.

 A38 (a).

The avascular necrosis rate is almost 100% with Hawkins type III and IV fractures.

 A39 (c).

Hawkins type I fractures are undisplaced. In type II injuries the fracture is displaced and there is subluxation or dislocation of the subtalar joint. In type III injuries there is dislocation of the body of the talus from both subtalar and ankle joints. In type IV injuries the talar head dislocates from the talonavicular joint. There is no type V with this classification.

 A40 (e).

With type III and IV injuries the avascular necrosis rate is 100%.

 A41 (d).

There is a 10% incidence of lumbar vertebral fracture and also of contralateral calcaneus fracture.

 A42 (c).

With fractures of the calcaneum, this angle is flattened.

 A43 (b).

The sural nerve passes down the posterolateral side of the leg and on to the dorsal aspect of the lateral side of the foot. At this point it is vulnerable to injury when approaching the lateral surface of the calcaneum.

A44   (a).

Therefore when performing internal fixation for Lisfranc fracture dislocations, a screw should connect the medial cuneiform to the second metatarsal base.

A45   (b).

The base of the second metatarsal is the keystone to the tarsometatarsal joint. The second metatarsal is longer and more recessed, which stabilises the tarsometatarsal joint. Therefore reducing the second metatarsal base is essential in order to achieve reduction of the whole tarsometatarsal complex.

Section 7

Shoulder and humerus

(Q1) What is the ratio of glenohumeral to scapulothoracic motion during shoulder abduction?

(a) 1:1.
(b) 1:2.
(c) 2:1.
(d) 1:3.
(e) 3:1.

(Q2) Injury to which of the following nerves results in winging of the scapula?

(a) Axillary nerve.
(b) Suprascapular nerve.
(c) Medial pectoral nerve.
(d) Thoracodorsal nerve.
(e) Long thoracic nerve.

(Q3) Which of the following nerves supplies the deltoid muscle?

(a) Axillary nerve.
(b) Suprascapular nerve.
(c) Medial pectoral nerve.
(d) Thoracodorsal nerve.
(e) Long thoracic nerve.

Q4   Which of the following nerves supplies the infraspinatus and supraspinatus muscles?

(a)   Axillary nerve.
(b)   Suprascapular nerve.
(c)   Medial pectoral nerve.
(d)   Thoracodorsal nerve.
(e)   Long thoracic nerve.

Q5   What is the relationship of the humeral head to the transcondylar axis of the distal humerus?

(a)   0–10° of anteversion.
(b)   10–20° of anteversion.
(c)   0–10° of retroversion.
(d)   10–20° of retroversion.
(e)   30–40° of retroversion.

Q6   Which of the following tendons does the transverse humeral ligament help to constrain?

(a)   Supraspinatus.
(b)   Short head of biceps.
(c)   Long head of biceps.
(d)   Coracobrachialis.
(e)   Subscapularis.

Q7   Which of the following structures is the most important dynamic stabiliser of the glenohumeral joint?

(a)   Glenoid labrum.
(b)   Posterior joint capsule.
(c)   Superior glenohumeral ligament.
(d)   Middle glenohumeral ligament.
(e)   Inferior glenohumeral ligament complex.

Q8   Which of the following is mainly responsible for supplying blood to the humeral head?

(a)   Anterior and posterior humeral circumflex arteries.
(b)   Subscapular artery.
(c)   Thoracodorsal artery.
(d)   Thoracoacromial artery.
(e)   Lateral thoracic artery.

Q9   Pain on cross-arm adduction indicates pathology at which of the following sites?

(a)   Glenohumeral joint.
(b)   Acromioclavicular joint.
(c)   Sternoclavicular joint.
(d)   Greater tuberosity.
(e)   Scapula body.

Q10   For which of the following muscles is the Gerber lift off test used to test function?

(a)   Supraspinatus.
(b)   Infraspinatus.
(c)   Teres minor.
(d)   Subscapularis.
(e)   Deltoid.

Q11   During the anterior approach to the shoulder, which of the following nerves is vulnerable to injury at the lower border of the subscapularis muscle?

(a)   Axillary nerve.
(b)   Suprascapular nerve.
(c)   Medial pectoral nerve.
(d)   Thoracodorsal nerve.
(e)   Long thoracic nerve.

(Q12) During the anterior approach to the shoulder, which of the following vascular structures provides a landmark to the interval between the deltoid and the pectoralis major?

(a) Axillary vein.
(b) Basilic vein.
(c) Cephalic vein.
(d) Axillary artery.
(e) Subscapular artery.

(Q13) During the anterior approach to the shoulder, which of the following arteries is most vulnerable to injury?

(a) Subclavian artery.
(b) Axillary artery.
(c) Subscapular artery.
(d) Thoracoacromial artery.
(e) Anterior humeral circumflex artery.

(Q14) A 35-year-old man complains of pain in the anterolateral part of his right shoulder. The pain troubles him at night, and he has difficulty performing overhead activities. On examination he is tender over the acromion and greater tuberosity. Shoulder range of motion is complete, but abduction is painful. Forward elevation and internal rotation of the shoulder reproduce his pain. What is the underlying diagnosis?

(a) Frozen shoulder.
(b) Anterior instability.
(c) Glenohumeral osteoarthritis.
(d) Subacromial impingement.
(e) Biceps tendon rupture.

(Q15) A 37-year-old woman gives a 2-week history of pain in the anterolateral aspect of her left shoulder. She has painful restriction of abduction. Radiographs demonstrate an area of calcification around the shoulder. Based on her symptoms, what is the most likely location of this calcification?

(a) Coracoacromial ligament.
(b) Subacromial bursa.
(c) Supraspinatus tendon.
(d) Infraspinatus tendon.
(e) Subscapularis tendon.

(Q16) What is the most appropriate first-line management in cases of acute calcific tendonitis?

(a) Non-steroidal anti-inflammatory drugs.
(b) Subacromial local anaesthetic injection.
(c) Subacromial local anaesthetic and steroid injection.
(d) Arthroscopic excision.
(e) Open excision.

(Q17) When performing an acromioplasty for impingement, in which of the following regions is it most important to resect?

(a) Anterior acromion.
(b) Posterior acromion.
(c) Medial acromion.
(d) Lateral acromion.
(e) Lateral clavicle.

(Q18) A 75-year-old man complains of pain and loss of function in his left shoulder. He is unable to abduct the shoulder, and cannot externally rotate the arm when held at his side in 90° of elbow flexion. Passively he allows full abduction and external rotation. Radiographs show superior migration of the humeral head, incongruity, articular erosion and subchondral collapse. What is the most likely underlying diagnosis?

(a) Septic arthritis.
(b) Rotator cuff arthropathy.
(c) Rheumatoid arthritis.
(d) Frozen shoulder.
(e) Supraspinatus tendon rupture.

Q19 A 24-year-old man, who is a keen weightlifter, complains of pain in his right shoulder. On examination he is tender over the acromioclavicular joint. Glenohumeral joint movements are complete and pain free. Radiographs show widening of the acromioclavicular joint with cystic changes. What is the underlying diagnosis?

(a) Supraspinatus tendon rupture.
(b) Bicipital tendinopathy.
(c) Clavicle fracture.
(d) Acromioclavicular joint osteoarthritis.
(e) Distal clavicular osteolysis.

Q20 What is the most common underlying mechanism of biceps tendinopathy?

(a) Frozen shoulder.
(b) Glenohumeral osteoarthritis.
(c) Instability.
(d) Subacromial impingement.
(e) Acromioclavicular joint separation.

Q21 In which of the following muscles is a tear associated with subluxation of the long head of biceps tendon?

(a) Infraspinatus.
(b) Supraspinatus.
(c) Teres minor.
(d) Subscapularis.
(e) Pectoralis major.

(Q22) What is the commonest location of osteophytes in gleno-humeral osteoarthritis?

(a) Superiorly on the humeral head.
(b) Inferiorly on the humeral head.
(c) Superiorly on the glenoid.
(d) Anteriorly on the glenoid.
(e) Posteriorly on the glenoid.

(Q23) In which of the following conditions is a humeral head replacement preferred to a total shoulder replacement?

(a) Glenohumeral osteoarthritis.
(b) Rheumatoid arthritis.
(c) Rotator cuff arthropathy.
(d) Avascular necrosis.
(e) Post-traumatic arthritis.

(Q24) During shoulder arthroplasty, which nerve is at risk if a coracoid osteotomy is performed?

(a) Musculocutaneous nerve.
(b) Axillary nerve.
(c) Suprascapular nerve.
(d) Long thoracic nerve.
(e) Lateral pectoral nerve.

(Q25) A 42-year-old woman who has diabetes mellitus complains of pain and stiffness in her right shoulder. On examination, she has significant restriction to passive movements in all directions. What is the underlying diagnosis?

(a) Glenohumeral osteoarthritis.
(b) Avascular necrosis.
(c) Septic arthritis.
(d) Subacromial impingement.
(e) Adhesive capsulitis.

Q26 Up to how long can it take to recover range of motion in cases of adhesive capsulitis, with non-operative management?

(a) 2–4 months.
(b) 4–6 months.
(c) 6–12 months.
(d) 12–18 months.
(e) 18–24 months.

Q27 What is the main risk associated with manipulation under anaesthesia for adhesive capsulitis?

(a) Dislocation.
(b) Axillary nerve injury.
(c) Axillary vein thrombosis.
(d) Humeral shaft fracture.
(e) Biceps tendon rupture.

Q28 A 25-year-old baseball pitcher complains of painful clicking and a popping sensation in his right dominant shoulder. He has a full range of motion in the shoulder, but the resisted supination external rotation test is positive. What is the most likely underlying diagnosis?

(a) Superior labral lesion.
(b) Long head of biceps tendon subluxation.
(c) Anterior instability.
(d) Posterior instability.
(e) Subacromial impingement.

 Q29 Which type of instability is more commonly seen in patients with epilepsy?

(a) Anterior.
(b) Posterior.
(c) Inferior.
(d) Superior.
(e) Multidirectional.

Q30   Which of the following best describes a Bankart lesion?

(a)   An impression fracture of the posterior humeral head.
(b)   An avulsion fracture of the greater tuberosity.
(c)   A detachment of the glenoid labrum.
(d)   An avulsion fracture of the lesser tuberosity.
(e)   A tear where the biceps tendon attaches to the superior labrum.

Q31   Which of the following factors is *not* associated with multidirectional instability?

(a)   No history of trauma.
(b)   Bilateral involvement.
(c)   Good response to rehabilitation.
(d)   May require an inferior capsular shift.
(e)   Bankart lesion.

Q32   Which of the following best describes a floating shoulder?

(a)   A fracture of the glenoid neck and body of the scapula.
(b)   A fracture of the glenoid neck and ipsilateral humeral neck.
(c)   A fracture of the clavicle and ipsilateral humeral neck.
(d)   A fracture of the glenoid neck and ipsilateral clavicle.
(e)   A fracture of the body of the scapula and ipsilateral humeral neck.

Q33   What anatomical abnormality occurs in type VI acromio-clavicular joint disruption?

(a)   Rupture of the acromioclavicular ligament.
(b)   Rupture of the coracoclavicular ligament.
(c)   Fracture of the distal clavicle.
(d)   Clavicle displaced into the trapezius muscle.
(e)   Clavicle displaced into the conjoined tendon.

(Q34) According to the Neer classification of proximal humeral fractures, which of the following is considered as displacement of a segment?

(a) 2 mm of translation.
(b) 5 mm of translation.
(c) 10° of angulation.
(d) 30° of angulation.
(e) 50° of angulation.

(Q35) A 45-year-old manual labourer is admitted to hospital with a displaced four-part proximal humerus fracture. What is the preferred method of treatment of this injury?

(a) Immobilisation in a collar and cuff for 8 weeks.
(b) Immobilisation in a hanging cast for 8 weeks.
(c) Minimal internal fixation with intramedullary pins.
(d) Open reduction and internal fixation with plate and screws.
(e) Prosthetic replacement.

(Q36) Dysfunction of which of the following nerves results from injury to the posterior cord of the brachial plexus?

(a) Radial nerve.
(b) Musculocutaneous nerve.
(c) Median nerve.
(d) Ulnar nerve.
(e) Suprascapular nerve.

(Q37) Which nerve is most commonly injured in humeral shaft fractures?

(a) Radial nerve.
(b) Musculocutaneous nerve.
(c) Median nerve.
(d) Ulnar nerve.
(e) Axillary nerve.

Which of the following constructs should be used when performing a plating of a fractured humeral shaft?

(a) Locking compression plate.
(b) Standard dynamic compression plate.
(c) Broad dynamic compression plate.
(d) One third tubular plate.
(e) Reconstruction plate.

 A 42-year-old man has sustained a minimally displaced spiral fracture at the junction of the middle and distal thirds of the humeral shaft. He has extensive bruising and swelling of the upper arm, but no open wound is present. He has loss of sensation over the first web space dorsally, and is unable to extend his wrist or fingers. What is the most appropriate management for this patient?

(a) Immediate manipulation under sedation.
(b) Urgent nerve conduction studies.
(c) A hanging plaster cast.
(d) Internal fixation and nerve exploration/repair.
(e) Internal fixation and tendon transfer.

 Prior to performing an open reduction and internal fixation of an isolated capitellum fracture, what is the most important factor that the patient should be warned about?

(a) Non-union rate.
(b) Risk of avascular necrosis.
(c) Risk of ulnar neuritis.
(d) Possibility of excision of the fragment.
(e) Wound infection.

Answers

A1 (c).

The shoulder moves approximately 180°, of which 120° is glenohumeral movement and 60° is scapulothoracic movement.

A2 (e).

The long thoracic nerve is derived from the ventral rami of C5, C6 and C7. It runs downward, passing either in front of or behind the middle scalene muscle. It then descends on to the anterior surface of the serratus anterior muscle, giving branches to supply it.

A3 (a).

The axillary nerve is derived from C5 and C6 nerve roots. It originates from the posterior cord of the brachial plexus. The axillary nerve innervates the teres minor and deltoid muscles, and supplies sensation to the regimental badge region. The axillary nerve is vulnerable to injury during anterior dislocation of the shoulder.

A4 (b).

The suprascapular nerve is derived from the upper trunk of the brachial plexus, typically receiving fibres from C5 and C6. It gives sensory branches to the glenohumeral and acromioclavicular joints, and supplies the supraspinatus and infraspinatus muscles.

A5 (e).

A6 (c).

The transverse humeral ligament is a broad band passing from the lesser to the greater tuberosity of the humerus. It converts the intertubercular groove into a canal, and restrains the long head of biceps tendon in this canal.

(e).

The inferior glenohumeral ligament is composed of an anterior and posterior band with an interposed axillary pouch. This complex is a major anterior stabiliser of the joint, especially with the arm abducted and externally rotated.

 (a).

The anterior and posterior humeral circumflex arteries arise from the axillary artery at the lower border of the subscapularis muscle. The posterior humeral circumflex artery runs backwards with the axillary nerve through the quadrangular space. The anterior humeral circumflex artery runs laterally across the neck of the humerus and eventually anastomoses with the posterior humeral circumflex artery.

 (b).

The cross-arm adduction test stresses the acromioclavicular joint and is useful for assessing pathology at this site.

- Chronopoulos E *et al.* Diagnostic value of physical tests for isolated chronic acromioclavicular lesions. *Am J Sports Med.* 2004; **32:** 655–61.

 (d).

The lift-off test was originally described by Gerber and Krushell in 1991. The patient is examined standing, and places their hand behind their back with the dorsum of the hand resting in the region of the mid-lumbar spine. The ability to actively lift the dorsum of the hand off the back constitutes a normal lift-off test. Inability to move the dorsum off the back constitutes an abnormal lift-off test and indicates subscapularis rupture or dysfunction.

 (a).

The axillary nerve lies initially behind the axillary artery, and in front of the subscapularis, and then passes downward to the lower border of the subscapularis. It winds backwards, along with the posterior humeral circumflex artery, passing through the quadrangular space. When dividing the subscapularis to approach the glenohumeral joint, only the superior seven-eighths of the muscle should be divided, in order to avoid injury to the axillary nerve.

(A12) (c).

In the upper third of the arm, the cephalic vein lies between the pectoralis major and the deltoid, and is accompanied by the deltoid branch of the thoracoacromial artery. It pierces the coracoclavicular fascia and, crossing the axillary artery, ends in the axillary vein just below the clavicle.

(A13) (e).

The anterior humeral circumflex artery runs horizontally, beneath the coracobrachialis and short head of the biceps brachii, in front of the neck of the humerus. On reaching the intertubercular sulcus, it gives off a branch which ascends in the sulcus to supply the head of the humerus and the shoulder joint. It is vulnerable to injury during its course across the anterior aspect of the humeral neck.

(A14) (d).

The clinical scenario is typical of subacromial impingement. Internal rotation with the shoulder and elbow flexed describes Hawkin's test, which is a very sensitive test for subacromial impingement.

- Park HB *et al.* Diagnostic accuracy of clinical tests for the different degrees of subacromial impingement syndrome. *J Bone Joint Surg Am.* 2005; **87**: 1446–55.
- Calis M *et al.* Diagnostic values of clinical diagnostic tests in subacromial impingement syndrome. *Ann Rheum Dis.* 2000; **59**: 44–7.

(A15) (c).

This woman is suffering from acute calcific tendonitis. The commonest location of a calcific deposit in this condition is the supraspinatus tendon.

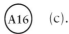 (c).

Around 80% of cases resolve with steroid and local anaesthetic injection followed by a course of physiotherapy.

 (a).

The anterior part of the acromion is most commonly the source of impingement, and therefore this must be adequately cleared. It is important not to excise the lateral part of the acromion, as this risks damaging the origin of the deltoid muscle.

(A18) (b).

This clinical scenario describes the typical findings of rotator cuff arthropathy. Rheumatoid arthritis may cause similar features, but the clinical scenario does not support this diagnosis. Although the supraspinatus tendon has ruptured, this in itself will not account for the extent of the symptoms and clinical findings.

(A19) (e).

Distal clavicular osteolysis is a condition that is related to repetitive microtrauma. It is common in athletes, and particularly in weight-lifters. In Cahill's paper, 44 of the 45 affected patients were weightlifters.

- Cahill BR. Osteolysis of the distal part of the clavicle in male athletes. *J Bone Joint Surg Am*. 1982; **64**: 1053–8.

(A20) (d).

There is a high incidence of biceps tendinopathy in patients with subacromial impingement. At arthroscopy, even though the biceps tendon may appear macroscopically normal, histopathological studies reveal evidence of inflammation in a high number of cases.

- Murthi AM *et al*. The incidence of pathologic changes of the long head of the biceps tendon. *J Shoulder Elbow Surg*. 2000; **9**: 382–5.

(A21)   (d).

An intact subscapularis muscle restrains the long head of biceps tendon in its anatomical location. A tear of the subscapularis results in loss of this restraint, and the long head of biceps tendon subluxes or dislocates. Subscapularis tears are associated with long head of biceps pathology in approximately 50% of cases.

- Tung GA *et al.* Subscapularis tendon tear: primary and associated signs on MRI. *J Comput Assist Tomogr.* 2001; **25**: 417–24.

(A22)   (b).

In glenohumeral osteoarthritis, osteophytes are most commonly seen on the inferior aspect of the humeral head.

(A23)   (c).

In the presence of rotator cuff arthropathy there is an increased risk of glenoid component failure. Therefore a total shoulder replacement is not preferred.

(A24)   (a).

The musculocutaneous nerve arises from the lateral cord of the brachial plexus, opposite the lower border of the pectoralis minor. It is derived from the fifth, sixth and seventh cervical nerves. It pierces the coracobrachialis muscle and passes obliquely between the biceps brachii and the brachialis, to the lateral side of the arm. Due to its close proximity to the coracobrachialis muscle, it is vulnerable to injury during a coracoid osteotomy or if the coracobrachialis is retracted forcefully.

(A25)   (e).

Adhesive capsulitis is characterised by a global restriction of passive movements. It is much more common in patients with diabetes.

(e).

It can take 18–24 months to recover range of motion with non-operative management. Manipulation under anaesthesia can reduce recovery time to 3–4 months. However, there may be an increased risk of dislocation, fracture, nerve palsy and rotator cuff tear with manipulation under anaesthesia.

- Noel E *et al.* Frozen shoulder. *Joint Bone Spine*. 2000; **67**: 393–400.
- Reichmister JP, Friedman SL. Long-term functional results after manipulation of the frozen shoulder. *Md Med J*. 1999; **48**: 7–11.

 (d).

There is an approximately 2% risk of a proximal humeral fracture with manipulation under anaesthesia. If there is any suspicion of this, image-intensifier films should be obtained.

- Hamdan TA, Al-Essa KA. Manipulation under anaesthesia for the treatment of frozen shoulder. *Int Orthop*. 2003; **27**: 107–9.

(A28) (a).

Superior labral anterior posterior (SLAP) lesions are common in athletes who participate in sports that involve throwing, such as baseball. The resisted supination external rotation test is highly specific and sensitive for SLAP lesions. With the patient lying supine, the shoulder is abducted to 90° and the forearm, which is in neutral rotation, is flexed to 70°. The patient supinates the forearm against resistance as the shoulder is gently externally rotated. Deep or anterior pain, clicking or reproduction of symptoms indicates a positive test.

- Myers TH *et al.* The resisted supination external rotation test. A new test for the diagnosis of superior labral anterior posterior lesions. *Am J Sports Med*. 2005; **33**: 1315–20.

(A29) (b).

In general, anterior instability is far more common than posterior instability. However, in patients with epilepsy, posterior and anterior instability occur with equal frequency. Thus posterior instability occurs much more commonly in epileptic patients than in the general population.

- Buhler M, Gerber C. Shoulder instability related to epileptic seizures. *J Shoulder Elbow Surg.* 2002; **11**: 339–44.

(A30) (c).

A Bankart lesion is a detachment of the glenoid labrum. (a) is a Hill-Sachs lesion and (e) is a SLAP lesion.

(A31) (e).

Patterns of instability can be remembered by using the mnemonics TUBS and AMBRI. TUBS = Traumatic Unidirectional Bankart lesion Surgery. AMBRI = Atraumatic Multidirectional Bilateral Rehabilitation Inferior capsular shift. From this it can be seen that a Bankart lesion is not typically associated with multidirectional instability.

(A32) (d).

Floating shoulder is an extremely rare injury, representing approximately 0.1% of all fractures. It results from high-energy trauma, and has a high incidence of associated injuries.

(A33) (e).

Rockwood *et al.* classified acromioclavicular joint dislocation into six subtypes. Type VI injuries are extremely rare, and result in rupture of the acromioclavicular ligament, joint capsule and coracoclavicular ligament. The clavicle is displaced into the tendons of the biceps and coracobrachialis.

(e).

According to the Neer classification, a fragment is displaced if more than 1 cm of translation occurs or more than 45° of angulation is present.

 (e).

Shoulder arthroplasty is a reliable technique for restoring function and comfort after three- or four-part fractures of the proximal humerus.

- Qian QR *et al.* Proximal humeral fractures treated with arthroplasty. *Chin J Traumatol.* 2005; **8**: 283–8.
- Dimakopoulos P *et al.* Hemiarthroplasty in the treatment of comminuted intra-articular fractures of the proximal humerus. *Clin Orthop Relat Res.* 1997; **341**: 7–11.

 (a).

The posterior cord gives rise to the radial and axillary nerves.

 (a).

Approximately 8% of humeral shaft fractures are associated with a radial nerve palsy. This occurs most commonly with middle and distal third fractures. Classically, the Holstein–Lewis fracture is associated with this complication. This is a fracture of the distal third of the humerus, where the radial nerve is caught between the bone ends when the fracture is reduced.

- Ekholm R *et al.* Fractures of the shaft of the humerus. An epidemiological study of 401 fractures. *J Bone Joint Surg Br.* 2006; **88**: 1469–73.

 (c).

A broad dynamic compression plate has the advantage of multi-planar screw placement, which prevents iatrogenic fracture.

(c).

In the vast majority of cases (90–100%), the radial nerve injury is a neuropraxia. Therefore there is no need for urgent exploration so long as there is no indication for internal fixation of the fracture. Nerve conduction studies should be performed 3 weeks after the injury to establish a baseline. If no recovery occurs by 4 months after the injury, the nerve should be explored.

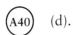 (d).

Capitellum fractures are classified into two morphological types – Hahn–Steinthal and Kocher–Lorenz. Hahn–Steinthal fractures involve a large part of the osseous portion of the capitellum, and may contain part of the adjacent lip of the trochlea. In Kocher–Lorenz fractures, the fragment is mainly composed of articular cartilage, with little bone attached. It is often impossible to determine the fracture type on the basis of imaging alone. In the case of Kocher–Lorenz fractures, it may be impossible to achieve adequate fixation of the fragment, and it may need to be excised. Therefore it is advisable to inform the patient of this possibility prior to surgery.

Section 8

Forearm and hand

Q1 The tendon of which muscle is found in the third dorsal extensor compartment?

(a) Extensor pollicis brevis.
(b) Extensor pollicis longus.
(c) Abductor pollicis longus.
(d) Extensor indicis proprius.
(e) Extensor carpi radialis longus.

Q2 Which muscles control the following movements of the ring finger: flexion at the metacarpophalangeal joints, interphalangeal joint extension and adduction?

(a) Flexor digitorum superficialis.
(b) Flexor digitorum profundus.
(c) Palmar interosseous.
(d) Dorsal interosseous.
(e) Lumbricals.

Q3 A 28-year-old construction worker sustains a crush injury to his little finger. Which of the following muscles will not be affected by such an injury?

(a) Flexor digitorum superficialis.
(b) Flexor digitorum profundus.
(c) Lumbricals.
(d) Palmar interosseous.
(e) Dorsal interosseous.

Q4 Which of the following structures is most medially located on the anterior aspect of the cubital fossa?

(a) Radial nerve.
(b) Brachial artery.
(c) Biceps tendon.
(d) Median nerve.
(e) Cephalic vein.

Q5 A lesion of the median nerve will result in paralysis of which of the following muscles?

(a) Lateral two lumbricals and opponens pollicis.
(b) Flexor carpi ulnaris and flexor digitorum profundus.
(c) Dorsal interossei and opponens pollicis.
(d) Medial two lumbricals and abductor pollicis brevis.
(e) Palmar interossei and medial two lumbricals.

Q6 A 32-year-old man complains of inability to hold a piece of paper between his index and middle fingers. Which of the following nerves is likely to have been injured?

(a) Median nerve.
(b) Radial nerve.
(c) Musculocutaneous nerve.
(d) Posterior interosseous nerve.
(e) Ulnar nerve.

Q7 Injury to the anterior interosseous nerve will result in paralysis of which of the following muscles?

(a) Flexor carpi ulnaris and pronator quadratus.
(b) Flexor pollicis longus and pronator quadratus.
(c) Flexor pollicis brevis and pronator quadratus.
(d) Flexor pollicis longus and opponens pollicis.
(e) Flexor digitorum profundus and opponens pollicis.

Q8   Which of the following structures does *not* pass through the carpal tunnel?

(a)   Flexor pollicis longus tendon.
(b)   Flexor digitorum profundus tendons.
(c)   Flexor carpi radialis tendon.
(d)   Median nerve.
(e)   Flexor digitorum superficialis tendons.

 Q9   A 22-year-old motorcyclist is involved in a road traffic accident. He sustains an injury to his left shoulder. On examination he is noted to have an internally rotated arm held by his side, with pronation of the forearm. He has sensory loss of the anterolateral aspect of the upper arm. Which nerve roots are damaged in this injury pattern?

(a)   C4,5.
(b)   C5,6.
(c)   C6,7.
(d)   C7,8.
(e)   C8,T1.

 Q10   How many annular pulleys are present in the hand?

(a)   1.
(b)   2.
(c)   3.
(d)   4.
(e)   5.

 Q11   With regard to flexor tendon function, which are the two most important pulleys?

(a)   A1 and A2.
(b)   C1 and C2.
(c)   C2 and C3.
(d)   A2 and A4.
(e)   A2 and A5.

A 44-year-old man is noted to have deformity of his left hand. He has flexion at the metacarpophalangeal joints, extension at the interphalangeal joints and adduction of the thumb. He has less passive interphalangeal joint flexion when the metacarpophalangeal joints are hyperextended than when they are flexed. What is the underlying diagnosis?

(a) Median nerve injury at the wrist.
(b) Ulnar nerve injury above the elbow.
(c) Ulnar nerve injury in the forearm.
(d) Intrinsic plus hand.
(e) Anterior interosseous nerve palsy.

 A traumatic boutonnière deformity corresponds to an extensor tendon injury in which zone?

(a) Zone I.
(b) Zone II.
(c) Zone III.
(d) Zone IV.
(e) Zone V.

 Which of the following best describes the characteristic deformities seen in rheumatoid arthritis affecting the hand and wrist?

(a) Carpus – volar, metacarpals – radial, digits – ulnar and volar.
(b) Carpus – dorsal, metacarpals – radial, digits – ulnar and volar.
(c) Carpus – volar, metacarpals – ulnar, digits – ulnar and volar.
(d) Carpus – volar, metacarpals – radial, digits – radial and dorsal.
(e) Carpus – dorsal, metacarpals – ulnar, digits – radial and volar.

(Q15) What is the main complication associated with caput ulnae syndrome?

(a) Weakness of wrist flexion.
(b) Extensor tendon rupture.
(c) Flexor tendon rupture.
(d) Ulnar deformity of the wrist.
(e) Paraesthesiae.

(Q16) In rheumatoid arthritis, rupture of the flexor pollicis longus tendon can occur due to attrition against a ridge on which of the following bones?

(a) Ulna.
(b) Trapezoid.
(c) Scaphoid.
(d) Trapezium.
(e) Capitate.

(Q17) Which tendon most commonly ruptures in patients with rheumatoid arthritis?

(a) Flexor pollicis longus.
(b) Flexor digitorum superficialis.
(c) Extensor digiti minimi.
(d) Extensor digitorum communis.
(e) Extensor pollicis longus.

(Q18) A 29-year-old man gives a 24-hour history of pain in his index finger. The finger is swollen and is held in a flexed position. It is very tender on palpation of the volar surface, and pain is exacerbated by passive extension of the finger. What is the underlying diagnosis?

(a) Felon.
(b) Paronychia.
(c) Flexor tendon rupture.
(d) Herpetic whitlow.
(e) Suppurative flexor tenosynovitis.

(Q19) Which of the following is *not* associated with a higher incidence of Dupuytren's contracture?

(a) Anglo-Saxon descent.
(b) Female sex.
(c) Epilepsy.
(d) Diabetes mellitus.
(e) Alcoholic cirrhosis.

(Q20) What is the commonest underlying inheritance pattern for Dupuytren's contracture?

(a) Sporadic.
(b) Autosomal recessive.
(c) Autosomal dominant.
(d) Sex-linked recessive.
(e) Sex-linked dominant.

(Q21) Which of the following surgical techniques for treating Dupuytren's contracture has the lowest rate of recurrence?

(a) Dermatofasciectomy.
(b) Fasciotomy.
(c) Total fasciectomy.
(d) Regional fasciectomy.
(e) Regional fasciectomy with the wound left open.

(Q22) Which of the following conditions is associated with Dupuytren's contracture?

(a) Plantar keratosis.
(b) Carpal tunnel syndrome.
(c) Trigger finger.
(d) Rotator cuff arthropathy.
(e) Peyronie's disease.

Q23 Which of the following is the commonest dissociation in volar intercalated segment instability?

(a) Scapholunate.
(b) Capitolunate.
(c) Scaphotrapezial.
(d) Lunotriquetral.
(e) Triquetrohamate.

 Q24 A 23-year-old mechanic has a 2-week history of pain and clicking in his right wrist. He sustained an injury to the wrist prior to the onset of symptoms, which he thought was just a sprain. On examination the wrist is swollen and he is diffusely tender over the dorsolateral part of the wrist. Standard radiographs of the wrist do not show any fracture, but dorsal translation of the capitate is noted. What should be the next investigation of choice?

(a) CT scan.
(b) MRI scan.
(c) Nuclear medicine bone scan.
(d) Ultrasound scan.
(e) Clenched-fist radiographs.

 Q25 A 36-year-old manual labourer complains of activity-related pain in his right dominant wrist. On examination he has mild swelling dorsally over the wrist. Grip strength is reduced, as is the arc of flexion and extension. Radiographs do not show any major abnormality, although negative ulnar variance is present. What is the most likely underlying diagnosis?

(a) Scapholunate dissociation.
(b) Kienbock's disease.
(c) Triangular fibrocartilage complex tear.
(d) Distal radio-ulnar joint instability.
(e) De Quervain's tenosynovitis.

(Q26) Which of the following upper limb deformities is *not* seen in patients with cerebral palsy?

(a) Elbow flexion.
(b) Forearm pronation.
(c) Wrist flexion.
(d) Finger flexion.
(e) Thumb abduction.

(Q27) During tension-band wiring of an olecranon fracture, which of the following structures is most at risk when inserting the longitudinal ulnar K-wires?

(a) Ulnar nerve.
(b) Posterior interosseous nerve.
(c) Anterior interosseous nerve.
(d) Brachial artery.
(e) Median nerve.

(Q28) A Bado grade II Monteggia fracture consists of a proximal ulna fracture and what abnormality of the radial head?

(a) Anterior dislocation.
(b) Posterior dislocation.
(c) Lateral dislocation.
(d) Medial dislocation.
(e) Radial shaft fracture.

(Q29) Which nerve is at risk of injury in Monteggia fractures?

(a) Ulnar nerve.
(b) Median nerve.
(c) Musculocutaneous nerve.
(d) Posterior interosseous nerve.
(e) Anterior interosseous nerve.

A 36-year-old woman fell from her bicycle and sustained a fracture to the shaft of her right radius. Radiographs demonstrated the fracture to be at the junction of the middle and distal thirds, and dislocation of the distal radio-ulnar joint was also noted. What type of injury pattern does this correspond to?

(a)   Galeazzi fracture.
(b)   Nightstick fracture.
(c)   Smith's fracture.
(d)   Essex–Lopresti fracture.
(e)   Monteggia fracture.

 A 45-year-old musician fell and sustained a comminuted, displaced fracture of his right dominant radial head. He is also tender over his right wrist. Radiographs do not show any fracture at the wrist, but the lateral view shows some subluxation at the distal radio-ulnar joint. Which of the following treatment options should ideally be avoided in this injury pattern?

(a)   Manipulation under anaesthesia.
(b)   Open reduction and internal fixation of the radial head.
(c)   Prosthetic replacement of the radial head.
(d)   Excision of the radial head.
(e)   Open reduction and internal fixation of the distal radio-ulnar joint.

 What specific complication can occur as a result of radiotherapy to treat heterotopic ossification encountered after elbow injury?

(a)   Anaemia.
(b)   Skin necrosis.
(c)   Axillary vein thrombosis.
(d)   Radiation-induced tumour.
(e)   Neuritis.

(Q33) What is the average radial inclination?

(a) 5°.
(b) 13°.
(c) 23°.
(d) 33°.
(e) 43°.

(Q34) Which of the following factors does *not* increase the risk of re-fracture after plate removal in internally fixed distal radius fractures?

(a) The use of large plates.
(b) Wound infection after plate removal.
(c) Plate removal less than 18 months after fracture.
(d) Plate removal without radiographic evidence of re-modelling.
(e) Failure to protect the forearm for 6 weeks after plate removal.

(Q35) Which of the following nerves is at risk when applying an external fixator for comminuted distal radial fractures?

(a) Recurrent branch of median nerve.
(b) Ulnar nerve.
(c) Anterior interosseous nerve.
(d) Posterior interosseous nerve.
(e) Superficial branch of radial nerve.

(Q36) Which type of scaphoid fracture carries the highest risk of avascular necrosis?

(a) Proximal pole fracture.
(b) Incomplete waist fracture.
(c) Complete waist fracture.
(d) Distal oblique fracture.
(e) Tuberosity fracture.

With ulnar collateral ligament injuries of the thumb meta-carpophalangeal joint, a Stener lesion occurs when the proximal part of the ligament is blocked by which of the following structures?

(a)   Abductor pollicis brevis.
(b)   Extensor pollicis longus.
(c)   Extensor pollicis brevis.
(d)   Adductor pollicis aponeurosis.
(e)   Abductor pollicis longus.

 Which of the following structures is not a component of the triangular fibrocartilage complex (TFCC)?

(a)   Ulnotriquetral ligament.
(b)   Ulnolunate ligament.
(c)   Flexor carpi ulnaris tendon sheath.
(d)   Radioulnar ligaments.
(e)   Ulnar collateral ligament.

 A 78-year-old woman sustained an undisplaced fracture of her distal radius, which was treated non-operatively with 6 weeks' immobilisation in a below-elbow cast. Two weeks after removal of the cast she complained of restricted finger movements. On examination, finger movement was slightly restricted but pain free. However, the woman was unable to lift up her thumb when her hand was placed flat on a table. What is the underlying diagnosis?

(a)   Complex regional pain syndrome.
(b)   Post-immobilisation stiffness.
(c)   Dorsal intercalated segment instability.
(d)   Ulnocarpal impingement.
(e)   Extensor pollicis longus rupture.

Q40 Which of the following factors is most important in guiding the management of metacarpal shaft fractures?

(a) Shortening.
(b) Malrotation.
(c) Angulation.
(d) Comminution.
(e) Mechanism of injury.

Answers

 A1 (b).

There are six extensor compartments on the dorsum of the hand: (1) abductor pollicis longus, extensor pollicis brevis; (2) extensor carpi radialis longus, extensor carpi radialis brevis; (3) extensor pollicis longus; (4) extensor indicis proprius, extensor digitorum communis; (5) extensor digiti quinti; (6) extensor carpi ulnaris.

 A2 (c).

The palmar interosseous muscles flex the metacarpophalangeal joint, extend the interphalangeal joint and adduct the fingers.

 A3 (e).

The little finger has no dorsal interosseous muscle.

 A4 (d).

The median nerve is the most medial structure traversing the cubital fossa.

 A5 (a).

The motor branch of the median nerve supplies the lumbricals to the index and middle fingers, the opponens pollicis and the abductor pollicis brevis.

(e).

The ulnar nerve supplies the palmar interosseous muscles, which are responsible for adduction of the fingers.

 (b).

The anterior interosseous nerve supplies the flexor digitorum profundus to the index and middle fingers, the flexor pollicis longus and the pronator quadratus.

 (c).

The carpal tunnel contains the median nerve and all the tendons that flex the fingers. The flexor carpi radialis tendon does not pass through the carpal tunnel.

 (b).

This clinical scenario describes Erb–Duchenne palsy, which results from damage to the C5 and C6 nerve roots.

 (e).

There are 8 pulleys in total in the hand – 5 annular pulleys and 3 cruciate pulleys. The pulleys are named A1–5 and C1–3.

 (d).

The A2 and A4 pulleys are relatively broad structures, which lie over the proximal and middle phalanges. It is important to preserve them in order to maintain optimal biomechanical function. In particular, the A4 pulley is biomechanically the most important pulley for maintaining independent interphalangeal joint function.

 (d).

This clinical scenario describes an intrinsic plus hand. This condition results from contracture or stiffness of the intrinsic muscles, and several underlying causes may be responsible. The Bunnell test has been described as a way of diagnosing tightness of the intrinsic muscles. If there is restricted passive interphalangeal joint flexion when the metacarpophalangeal joints are extended compared with when they are flexed, the intrinsic muscles are tight.

(A13) (c).

Zone III for extensor tendon injuries corresponds to the proximal interphalangeal joint. In a traumatic boutonnière deformity, rupture of the central slip of the extensor tendon occurs at the proximal interphalangeal joint. This results in flexion at the proximal interphalangeal joint and compensatory hyperextension at the distal interphalangeal joint.

(A14) (a).

In rheumatoid arthritis, there is volar migration of the carpus and radial deviation of the metacarpals. The digits translate in an ulnar and volar direction.

(A15) (b).

In caput ulnae syndrome, dorsal subluxation of the distal ulna occurs with supination of the carpus. Caput ulnae syndrome is most commonly seen in patients with rheumatoid arthritis. Weakness of the extensor tendons already exists due to the extensive synovitis seen in rheumatoid arthritis. Attrition of these weakened extensor tendons over the prominent ulnar head can lead to rupture of the tendons, resulting in dropped digits.

(A16) (d).

Synovitis, which occurs in rheumatoid arthritis, results in weakening of the tendons. The flexor pollicis longus tendon can rupture as a result of attrition against a bony ridge found on the trapezium.

(A17) (c).

The extensor digiti minimi usually ruptures first, but rupture may go unnoticed because the extensor digitorum communis extends all four fingers simultaneously.

- Williamson L *et al.* Screening for extensor tendon rupture in rheumatoid arthritis. *Rheumatology (Oxford).* 2001; **40**: 420–3.

(e).

This clinical scenario describes an infection of the flexor tendon sheath. Kanavel described four cardinal signs of infectious tenosynovitis: (1) swelling along the entire flexor surface; (2) tenderness over the course of the tendon sheath; (3) pain on passive extension of the finger; (4) an inability to straighten the finger at rest.

 (b).

Approximately 70% of cases of Dupuytren's contracture occur in men.

- Geoghegan JM *et al.* Dupuytren's disease risk factors. *J Hand Surg Br.* 2004; **29:** 423–6.

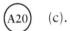 (c).

Dupuytren's contracture appears to follow an autosomal dominant model of inheritance. It remains unclear whether there is a genetic basis for the many seemingly sporadic cases.

- Burge P. Genetics of Dupuytren's disease. *Hand Clin.* 1999; **15:** 63–71.

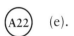 (a).

Significantly lower recurrence rates are reported with dermatofasciectomy compared with fasciectomy in Dupuytren's disease. Therefore dermatofasciectomy should be the procedure of choice for patients with aggressive disease.

- Armstrong JR *et al.* Dermofasciectomy in the management of Dupuytren's disease. *J Bone Joint Surg Br.* 2000; **82:** 90–4.

(A22) (e).

Peyronie's disease, which is characterised by fibrosis and curvature of the penis, is associated with Dupuytren's disease. Approximately 5–10% of patients with Dupuytren's contracture may also suffer from Peyronie's disease.

(A23)   (d).

Lunotriquetral dissociation is the commonest cause of volar intercalated segment instability. Scapholunate dissociation causes dorsal intercalated segment instability. The other dissociations listed do cause volar intercalated segment instability, but much less commonly than does lunotriquetral dissociation.

(A24)   (e).

In the absence of a fracture, the most likely injury is to the scapholunate ligament. Clenched-fist radiographs should demonstrate the presence of scapholunate dissociation. However, if these are normal and clinical suspicion is still high, an MRI scan should be performed.

(A25)   (b).

This clinical scenario gives a history typical of Kienbock's disease. Negative ulnar variance has also been associated with Kienbock's disease. A recent meta-analysis demonstrated that the odds ratio for developing Kienbock's disease was 3.10 times higher in individuals with negative ulnar variance compared with individuals with positive or neutral variance. However, this finding was not statistically significant.

- Chung KC *et al*. Is negative ulnar variance a risk factor for Kienbock's disease? A meta-analysis. *Ann Plast Surg*. 2001; 47: 494–9.

(A26)   (e).

All of the deformities listed are commonly seen in cerebral palsy. However, thumb abduction is not seen. In fact, the thumb in palm deformity is typically seen.

(A27)   (c).

The anterior interosseous nerve is at risk of injury if the K-wires are inserted too far through the anterior ulnar cortex.

(b).

Anterior dislocation of the radial head occurs in a Bado grade I Monteggia fracture. In a grade II fracture, posterior dislocation of the radial head is seen. In a grade III injury, lateral dislocation occurs. In grade IV injuries, a fracture of the proximal radius occurs in addition to the proximal ulna fracture. Medial dislocation is not described in the Bado classification.

 (d).

The posterior interosseous nerve is at risk of injury in Monteggia fractures. This may occur as an acute or delayed event.

- Holst-Nielsen F, Jensen V. Tardy posterior interosseous nerve palsy as a result of an unreduced radial head dislocation in Monteggia fractures: a report of two cases. *J Hand Surg Am.* 1984; **9**: 572–5.
- Yamamoto K *et al.* Posterior interosseous nerve palsy as a complication of Monteggia fractures. *Nippon Geka Hokan.* 1977; **46**: 46–56.

 (a).

A Galeazzi fracture occurs when the radial shaft is fractured along with disruption of the distal radio-ulnar joint. This is an unstable injury, which always requires open reduction and internal fixation (ORIF).

 (d).

This clinical scenario is typical of an Essex–Lopresti fracture. In this injury a fracture of the radial head occurs, along with disruption of the distal radio-ulnar joint and interosseous membrane. Ideally, open reduction and internal fixation of the radial head should be performed. If, due to extensive comminution, this is not possible then prosthetic replacement should be undertaken. Excision of the radial head should be avoided, as this causes proximal migration of the radius, which results in elbow and wrist pain due to ulnocarpal impingement.

(A32) (e).

Neuritis is a potential complication following radiotherapy to treat heterotopic ossification around the elbow. Axillary vein thrombosis has been reported with a combination of chemotherapy and radiotherapy. For treating heterotopic ossification, only a single shot of radiotherapy is given, and therefore malignant change is very unlikely.

(A33) (c).

The average radial inclination is 23°, with a range of 15–30°.

(A34) (b).

Wound infection after removal of metalwork has not been linked to an increased risk of re-fracture. However, all of the other factors listed do increase the risk of re-fracture after plate removal.

(A35) (e).

The superficial branch of the radial nerve is at risk of injury at the time of proximal pin insertion.

(A36) (a).

The scaphoid is supplied by the radial artery. The most important vascular branches enter the scaphoid through foraminae along its dorsal ridge, just distal to the waist. The proximal pole is supplied in a retrograde fashion. In proximal pole fractures, the blood supply is disrupted, rendering the proximal fragment susceptible to avascular necrosis.

(A37) (d).

In a Stener lesion, a distal rupture of the thumb ulnar collateral ligament occurs at the thumb metacarpophalangeal joint, with interposition of the adductor pollicis aponeurosis between the distal site of attachment of the ruptured ligament and the detached ligament. The interposed adductor aponeurosis maintains separation between the ruptured ends of the ligament, and thus prevents ligamentous healing and restoration of joint stability.

(c).

The tendon sheath of extensor carpi ulnaris is a component of the TFCC, but not the tendon sheath of flexor carpi ulnaris.

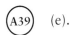 (e).

This clinical scenario describes rupture of the extensor pollicis longus tendon. This is a well-recognised complication following fracture of the distal radius. The fracture produces irregularity over the dorsal surface of the distal radius, which can result in attrition rupture of the tendon. Rupture of the extensor pollicis longus tendon usually occurs just distal to Lister's tubercle. The treatment of choice is an extensor indicis proprius tendon transfer.

- Orljanski W *et al*. Rupture of the extensor pollicis longus tendon after wrist trauma. *Acta Chir Plast*. 2002; **44:** 129–31.

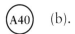 (b).

Any clinical malrotation cannot be tolerated, as it will interfere with hand function, due to an inability to clench the fist. Therefore rotational deformities resulting from metacarpal fractures require correction.

Section 9

Spine

(Q1) Which of the following cervical vertebrae does not have a bifid spinous process?

(a) C3.
(b) C4.
(c) C5.
(d) C6.
(e) C7.

(Q2) The vertebral artery typically enters the spine via the transverse foramen of which of the following vertebrae?

(a) C3.
(b) C4.
(c) C5.
(d) C6.
(e) C7.

(Q3) Which of the following cervical nerves exit the spinal canal posterior to the facet joints?

(a) C2.
(b) C3.
(c) C4.
(d) C5.
(e) C6.

Q4 Which of the following tracts is responsible for transmitting pain and temperature sensation?

(a) Dorsal columns.
(b) Lateral spinothalamic tract.
(c) Anterior spinothalamic tract.
(d) Lateral corticospinal tract.
(e) Anterior corticospinal tract.

Q5 Which of the following nerve roots is responsible for middle finger sensation?

(a) C3.
(b) C4.
(c) C5.
(d) C6.
(e) C7.

Q6 Which of the following nerve roots is responsible for wrist extension?

(a) C3.
(b) C4.
(c) C5.
(d) C6.
(e) C7.

Q7 In the neck, to which of the following levels does the thyroid cartilage correspond?

(a) C2–3.
(b) C3–4.
(c) C4–5.
(d) C5–6.
(e) C6–7.

Q8 An absent ankle jerk indicates involvement of which of the following nerve roots?

(a) L2.
(b) L3.
(c) L4.
(d) L5.
(e) S1.

Q9 Involvement of which of the following nerve roots is indicated by weakness of the extensor hallucis longus?

(a) L2.
(b) L3.
(c) L4.
(d) L5.
(e) S1.

Q10 Lhermitte's sign results in pain and electric shock-like sensations in the limbs with which of the following?

(a) Neck flexion.
(b) Neck rotation.
(c) Axial compression of the neck.
(d) Neck traction.
(e) Neck extension.

Q11 Which of the following features is *not* typically associated with cervical myelopathy?

(a) Positive Hoffman's sign.
(b) Positive Spurling's test.
(c) Positive plantar reflex.
(d) Inverted radial reflex.
(e) Finger escape sign.

Q12 Which of the following is the commonest type of disc herniation?

(a) Central.
(b) Paracentral.
(c) Foraminal.
(d) Extraforaminal.
(e) Sequestrated.

Q13 What proportion of patients who experience a second episode of sciatica will go on to experience a third episode?

(a) 10%.
(b) 25%.
(c) 50%.
(d) 75%.
(e) 90%.

Q14 Which of the following statements about lumbar disc herniation is *not* true?

(a) Around 80–90% of patients will improve with non-operative management.
(b) Surgical intervention does not increase the likelihood of recovery from neurological deficit.
(c) After surgery, approximately 30% of patients have residual sensory deficit despite relief of pain.
(d) After surgery, there is a 5% chance of recurrent disc herniation at the same level.
(e) Small disc extrusions have a greater likelihood of total spontaneous resorption.

Q15 A 75-year-old man complains of pain in his buttocks and the back of his legs. The pain is exacerbated by walking and is relieved by leaning forward. What is the most likely underlying diagnosis?

(a) Spondylolisthesis.
(b) Sciatica.

(c) Cauda equina syndrome.

(d) Spinal stenosis.

(e) Piriformis syndrome.

Q16 Absolute spinal stenosis is present when the anteroposterior dimension of the spinal canal falls below which of the following values?

(a) 20 mm.

(b) 18 mm.

(c) 15 mm.

(d) 10 mm.

(e) 5 mm.

Q17 Which of the following factors is not associated with a higher incidence of cervical spine involvement in patients with rheumatoid arthritis?

(a) Cigarette smoking.

(b) Rheumatoid factor positive.

(c) Regular corticosteroid use.

(d) Male sex.

(e) Multiple joint involvement.

Q18 Which of the following biochemical changes does *not* occur with lumbar disc degeneration?

(a) Increased levels of collagen type I.

(b) Decreased water content.

(c) Decreased fibronectin content.

(d) Decreased proteoglycan content.

(e) Increased matrix metalloproteinases.

Q19 Which of the following statements about spondylolysis is *not* true?

(a) It can be unilateral or bilateral.

(b) It may be congenital.

(c) It is more common among Inuit people.

(d)   An underlying genetic predisposition is present.
(e)   There is an increased incidence among individuals who engage in sports that hyperextend the spine.

Q20   Which of the following nerve roots is most commonly compressed in isthmic spondylolisthesis?

(a)   L2.
(b)   L3.
(c)   L4.
(d)   L5.
(e)   S1.

Q21   Which of the following statements about degenerative spondylolisthesis is *not* true?

(a)   It corresponds to type III according to the Wiltse classification.
(b)   It is more common in women.
(c)   It is more common in African-Americans.
(d)   It most commonly occurs at the L4–5 level.
(e)   It is associated with coronally orientated facet joints.

Q22   Which of the following factors is *not* associated with an increased risk of slip progression in spondylolisthesis?

(a)   Male sex.
(b)   Slip angles greater than 10°.
(c)   High-grade slips.
(d)   Young age at presentation.
(e)   Type I slips.

Q23   Which of the following statements about vertebral osteo-myelitis is *not* true?

(a)   The commonest causative organism is *Staphylococcus aureus*.
(b)   The lumbar spine is the commonest site of involve-ment.

(c) Indium-labelled leucocyte scans are highly sensitive for diagnosis.

(d) In children, bacterial emboli are deposited in the nucleus pulposus.

(e) Up to 75% of patients respond to parenteral antibiotics.

Q24 Which of the following statements about epidural abscess is correct?

(a) The commonest causative organism is *Staphylococcus epidermidis*.

(b) It most commonly affects the thoracic spine.

(c) It is most commonly located posteriorly in the spine.

(d) MRI with gadolinium is the investigation of choice.

(e) In the absence of neurology it is acceptable to manage it non-operatively.

Q25 Which of the following abnormalities is present in Brown-Sequard syndrome?

(a) Loss of contralateral motor function and ipsilateral pain and temperature sensation.

(b) Loss of ipsilateral motor function and contralateral pain and temperature sensation.

(c) Loss of contralateral motor function and ipsilateral proprioception and vibration sensation.

(d) Loss of contralateral fine touch sensation and ipsilateral pain and temperature sensation.

(e) Loss of contralateral fine motor function and ipsilateral pain and temperature sensation.

Q26 Which of the following factors is *not* associated with an increased incidence of non-union of axis fractures?

(a) Extensive comminution.

(b) Greater than 6 mm displacement.

(c) Delay in diagnosis.

(d) Female sex.

(e) Treatment in a halo vest.

Which of the following is an accurate description of a hangman's fracture?

(a)   A fracture of the spinous process of C7.
(b)   A fracture through the body of C3.
(c)   A fracture of the anterior and posterior arch of C1.
(d)   A fracture through the body of C2.
(e)   A fracture through both pars interarticularis of C2.

 At what level does the spinal cord typically end?

(a)   T12.
(b)   L1.
(c)   L2.
(d)   L4.
(e)   L5.

 Which of the following statements about cervical facet joint dislocations is true?

(a)   A unilateral dislocation results in 50% subluxation of the vertebral body.
(b)   A bilateral dislocation results in 25% subluxation of the vertebral body.
(c)   Axial traction should never be applied in awake patients.
(d)   Closed reduction is rarely successful.
(e)   Unilateral dislocations are associated with a higher incidence of nucleus pulposus herniation.

 Which of the following is *not* true of Chance fractures?

(a)   They most commonly occur as a result of a flexion–distraction injury.
(b)   They are associated with the use of lap seat belts.
(c)   Up to 50% of patients may have concomitant abdominal injuries.
(d)   They most commonly occur in the thoracolumbar region.

(e)   A Chance fracture is an unstable injury which should always be managed with open reduction and internal fixation.

Answers

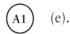 (e).

The two upper cervical vertebrae are atypical. The vertebrae from C3–6 have a bifid spinous process. C7 is known as the vertebra prominens, and although it has a long spinous process it is not bifid.

 (d).

The vertebral artery is the first branch of the subclavian artery. It ascends through the foramina in the transverse processes of the upper six cervical vertebrae. Then it winds behind the superior articular process of the atlas and enters the skull through the foramen magnum.

 (a).

In general, cervical nerves exit the spinal canal anterior to the facet joints. However, the C2 nerves exit posterior to the facet joints.

 (b).

The lateral spinothalamic tract transmits pain and temperature sensation. The dorsal columns transmit proprioception and vibration. The lateral corticospinal tract transmits ipsilateral motor signals, and the anterior spinothalamic tract transmits contralateral light touch. The anterior corticospinal tract is responsible for fine motor control.

 (e).

In the hand, the thumb is supplied by C6, the index, middle and ring fingers by C7, and the little finger by C8.

A6 (d).

C6 is the myotome responsible for elbow flexion and wrist extension.

A7 (c).

The thyroid cartilage is the largest cartilage of the larynx. It lies at the C4–5 level. The cricoid cartilage lies opposite C6.

A8 (e).

L5 is the myotome responsible for extension of the hallux. S1 controls plantar flexion of the foot, and an absent ankle jerk signifies pathology of the S1 nerve root.

A9 (d).

The L5 nerve root is responsible for innervation of the extensor hallucis longus. Weakness of big toe extension signifies pathology of the L5 nerve roots.

A10 (a).

Lhermitte's sign refers to a sudden electric shock-like sensation down the neck and back, triggered by neck flexion. This was originally described in a patient with multiple sclerosis and dorsal column dysfunction. However, Lhermitte's sign also occurs in cervical spondylosis, cervical disc herniation and myelopathy.

A11 (b).

Spurling's test is positive when neck extension and lateral rotation cause pain on the ipsilateral side. This test is indicative of an underlying radiculopathy. Unlike the other tests listed, it is not associated with cervical myelopathy.

A12 (b).

Paracentral or posterolateral disc herniation is the commonest type seen.

A13 (c).

Approximately 50% of patients who experience a second episode of sciatica go on to develop a further episode.

A14 (e).

Large disc extrusions have a greater likelihood of total spontaneous resorption.

A15 (d).

This clinical scenario is typical of patients with spinal stenosis. This condition results from narrowing of the spinal canal, which causes nerve root or cord compression, leading to persistent pain in the buttocks, limping, lack of sensation in the lower extremities, and decreased physical activity.

A16 (d).

Absolute spinal stenosis occurs when the anteroposterior dimension of the spinal canal falls below 10 mm. Relative spinal stenosis is said to occur when the measurement is 10–12 mm. This can be measured on plain films. However, a CT or MRI scan will allow more accurate measurement of the mid-sagittal canal diameter. It also enables measurement of the cross-sectional area of the canal. Absolute spinal stenosis is said to occur when the canal cross-sectional area falls below 100 mm^2.

A17 (a).

Cigarette smoking has been implicated as a risk factor for developing lower back pain. However, there is no evidence that it increases the likelihood of cervical spine involvement in patients with rheumatoid arthritis.

A18 (c).

The amount of fibronectin actually increases during lumbar disc degeneration. Fibronectin has been shown to down-regulate aggrecan synthesis but to up-regulate the production of some matrix metalloproteinases in *in-vitro* systems.

A19 (b).

No congenital cases have been reported to date. The current thinking is that it is a developmental condition. An underlying genetic predisposition may be present, as the incidence is increased by fourfold in first-degree relatives.

A20 (d).

Isthmic spondylolisthesis most commonly occurs at the L5–S1 level. However, the upper exiting nerve roots are compressed, as opposed to the lower traversing nerve roots.

A21 (e).

Degenerative spondylolisthesis is associated with sagitally orientated facet joints rather than coronally orientated facet joints.

A22 (a).

Female sex is associated with an increased risk of slip progression in spondylolisthesis.

A23 (c).

Indium-labelled leucocyte scanning is not sensitive for the diagnosis of vertebral osteomyelitis.

- Palestro CJ *et al.* Radionuclide diagnosis of vertebral osteomyelitis: indium-111-leukocyte and technetium-99m-methylene diphosphonate bone scintigraphy. *J Nucl Med.* 1991; **32**: 1861–5.

MRI with gadolinium enhancement is the investigation of choice.

- Tehranzadeh J *et al.* Magnetic resonance imaging of osteomyelitis. *Crit Rev Diagn Imaging.* 1992; **33**: 495–534.

A24 (e).

In the absence of neurological symptoms an epidural abscess can be managed non-operatively. However, a protracted course of antibiotics is required. Initially intravenous antibiotics should be given, and if a satisfactory response is observed, conversion to oral antibiotics can take place. Duration of therapy is guided by measurement of inflammatory markers, such as ESR and CRP.

 (b).

Brown-Sequard syndrome results from hemisection of the spine, although it is rarely seen in clinical practice. Interruption of the lateral corticospinal tracts, the lateral spinothalamic tract and at times the dorsal columns produces a picture of a spastic weak leg with brisk reflexes, and a strong contralateral leg with loss of pain and temperature sensation.

 (d).

There is no effect of patient gender on the union of axis fractures.

 (e).

A hangman's fracture results from a severe extension injury – for example, from an automobile accident in which the face forcibly strikes the dashboard, or from hanging. This type of fracture consists of bilateral pars fractures of the C2 vertebral body. Associated anterior subluxation or dislocation of the C2 vertebral body is also seen.

 (b).

Typically the spinal cord ends at the level of the L1 vertebra.

 (e).

Unilateral facet joint dislocations carry double the risk of nucleus pulposus herniation compared with bilateral facet joint dislocations (26% compared with 13%).

A30 (e).

A Chance fracture is a pure bony injury extending from posterior to anterior, through the spinous process, pedicles and vertebral body. The typical history is of a rear-seat passenger wearing a lap seat belt, involved in a road traffic accident. In general, Chance fractures can be managed by immobilisation in a thoracolumbosacral orthosis (TLSO) or hyperextension cast. Surgical indications include the polytraumatised patient, significant displacement, or patients whose size makes closed treatment difficult or impractical.

Section 10

Orthopaedic oncology

Q1 Which of the following statements about unicameral bone cysts is true?

    (a) They most commonly occur in men aged 20–30 years.
    (b) They are most commonly located in the distal humerus.
    (c) Closed treatment should not be implemented in pathological fractures through a unicameral bone cyst.
    (d) Intracystic steroid injection is contraindicated.
    (e) Intracystic bone-marrow injection is an accepted treatment option.

Q2 Which of the following statements about aneurysmal bone cysts (ABCs) is *not* true?

    (a) ABCs most commonly occur during the second decade of life.
    (b) ABCs are benign expansile cystic lesions.
    (c) ABCs can be rapidly growing destructive lesions.
    (d) Radiotherapy is the treatment of choice.
    (e) There is a high incidence of accompanying tumours associated with ABCs.

Q3 Which of the following statements about aneurysmal bone cysts (ABCs) is true?

    (a) ABCs most commonly occur in the distal radius.
    (b) ABCs most commonly occur in the diaphysis.
    (c) ABCs are more common in men.

(d)   Liquid nitrogen is contraindicated as adjuvant therapy.
(e)   Radiographs demonstrate a 'soap-bubble' appearance.

Q4   A 24-year-old man complains of pain in his right lower leg. The pain is exacerbated by activity and is worse at night. It is significantly improved by taking aspirin. What is the most likely underlying diagnosis?

(a)   Osteoid osteoma.
(b)   Osteosarcoma.
(c)   Chondroblastoma.
(d)   Stress fracture.
(e)   Giant-cell tumour.

Q5   Which of the following statements about osteoid osteoma is *not* true?

(a)   Spinal osteoid osteoma may induce a painful scoliosis.
(b)   Osteoid osteoma is characteristically associated with significant systemic symptoms.
(c)   Occasional spontaneous regression has been reported.
(d)   Radiographs typically demonstrate a nidus less than 2 cm in diameter, surrounded by a zone of sclerosis.
(e)   Osteoid osteomata produce high levels of prosta-glandin E_2.

Q6   Which of the following is the commonest primary bone tumour found in the hand?

(a)   Giant-cell tumour.
(b)   Aneurysmal bone cyst.
(c)   Enchondroma.
(d)   Osteoid osteoma.
(e)   Osteochondroma.

Which of the following statements about adamantinoma is true?

(a) Adamantinoma is a high-grade malignant tumour of mesodermal origin.
(b) The commonest site of involvement is the pelvis.
(c) Adamantinoma is highly radiosensitive.
(d) Areas of osteofibrous dysplasia may give rise to adamantinoma.
(e) Metastatic involvement of the lungs does not occur.

 A 9-year-old girl is seen in the emergency department after having sustained a fracture of the right distal femur. Radiographs show fracture through an abnormal area of bone. On closer questioning, the girl complains of recurrent pains in her other limbs. Radiographs show multiple lesions in other bones. On examination, the girl is found to have numerous café-au-lait spots on her body and is under investigation for precocious puberty. What is the most likely underlying diagnosis?

(a) Ollier's disease.
(b) Maffucci syndrome.
(c) Multiple myeloma.
(d) Ewing's sarcoma.
(e) McCune–Albright syndrome.

 Which of the following statements about fibrous dysplasia is *not* true?

(a) The condition is usually monostotic.
(b) The condition improves during pregnancy.
(c) The lesions are typically located in the diaphysis or metaphysis.
(d) Autosomal dominant inheritance is seen in a minority of cases.
(e) Radiographs typically demonstrate no periosteal reaction.

Q10   Which of the following tumours can metastasise to the lungs?

(a)   Chondroblastoma.
(b)   Enchondroma.
(c)   Osteoid osteoma.
(d)   Osteochondroma.
(e)   Osteoblastoma.

Q11   Which of the following is the commonest skeletal neoplasm?

(a)   Enchondroma.
(b)   Osteosarcoma.
(c)   Osteochondroma.
(d)   Giant-cell tumour.
(e)   Chondroblastoma.

Q12   Which of the following statements about osteochondroma is *not* true?

(a)   Approximately 40% of lesions occur around the knee.
(b)   It more commonly occurs in males.
(c)   It only occurs in bones that develop from endochondral ossification.
(d)   The lesions continue to increase in size after growth plate closure.
(e)   Osteochondroma has been reported to occur after radiotherapy.

Q13   What is the risk of malignant transformation for a solitary osteochondroma?

(a)   Less than 1%.
(b)   5%.
(c)   10%.
(d)   15%.
(e)   20%.

(Q14) Which of the following statements about hereditary multiple osteochondromatosis is true?

(a) The condition is inherited in an autosomal recessive manner.
(b) It most commonly occurs in the second decade of life.
(c) The risk of malignant transformation is approximately 1%.
(d) Pedunculated lesions carry a higher risk of malignant transformation.
(e) A cartilage cap measuring 1–6 mm in diameter is normally present.

(Q15) Which of the following statements about chondrosarcoma is true?

(a) Peak incidence occurs in the first and second decades of life.
(b) There is an equal incidence among males and females.
(c) There is an increased incidence in Ollier's disease.
(d) Clear-cell chondrosarcoma carries a worse prognosis.
(e) There is a 50% survival rate in dedifferentiated chondrosarcoma.

(Q16) A 15-year-old boy has a 6-week history of pain and swelling in his left thigh. There is no history of trauma prior to the onset of symptoms. He has also been suffering from intermittent fevers. Blood tests reveal anaemia, leucocytosis and a raised ESR. Radiographs of the femur demonstrate a central lytic lesion with a lamellated 'onion-skin' periosteal reaction. Cytogenetic tests reveal the presence of a t (11;22) translocation. What is the most likely underlying diagnosis?

(a) Osteosarcoma.
(b) Ewing's sarcoma.
(c) Chondrosarcoma.
(d) Rhabdomyosarcoma.
(e) Osteomyelitis.

Q17 Which of the following statements about Ewing's sarcoma is true?

(a) It occurs more commonly in African-Americans.
(b) It most commonly occurs during the fifth decade of life.
(c) It most commonly occurs in the tibia.
(d) There is an equal incidence in men and women.
(e) It originates from cells of the neural crest.

Q18 In which of the following conditions does secondary fibro-sarcoma *not* arise?

(a) Paget's disease.
(b) Chronic osteomyelitis.
(c) Fibrous dysplasia.
(d) Osteoid osteoma.
(e) Irradiated giant-cell tumour.

Q19 Which of the following is the commonest primary malignant tumour of bone?

(a) Osteosarcoma.
(b) Fibrosarcoma.
(c) Chondrosarcoma.
(d) Ewing's sarcoma.
(e) Malignant fibrous histiocytoma.

Q20 At which of the following sites is osteosarcoma most commonly found?

(a) Proximal humerus.
(b) Proximal tibia.
(c) Distal femur.
(d) Pelvis.
(e) Radius.

(Q21) Which of the following variants of osteosarcoma is most commonly associated with pathological fracture?

(a) Osteoblastic.
(b) Telangiectatic.
(c) Multifocal.
(d) Parosteal.
(e) Periosteal.

(Q22) Which of the following laboratory tests is of most prognostic value in the assessment of osteosarcoma?

(a) C-reactive protein.
(b) Erythrocyte sedimentation rate.
(c) Aspartate aminotransferase.
(d) Alanine aminotransferase.
(e) Alkaline phosphatase.

(Q23) With regard to open biopsy of musculoskeletal tumours, which of the following statements is *not* true?

(a) Transverse incisions are contraindicated.
(b) A frozen-section sample of biopsy specimen should always be analysed.
(c) The shortest route to the lesion that does not violate more than one compartment should be used.
(d) If a drain is used, it should be placed lateral to the incision.
(e) The biopsy tract should be as remote as possible from the neurovascular bundle.

(Q24) From which of the following sites do primary tumours rarely metastasise to bone?

(a) Ovary.
(b) Breast.
(c) Kidney.
(d) Prostate.
(e) Lung.

A 68-year-old woman, who is known to have metastatic breast cancer, complains of severe pain in her right upper arm. Radiographs demonstrate a lytic lesion of the proximal humerus, with 50% cortical destruction. What is the Mirels' score for this patient?

    (a) 4.
    (b) 6.
    (c) 8.
    (d) 9.
    (e) 11.

Answers

 (e).

Intracystic bone-marrow injection has yielded good results in the treatment of unicameral bone cysts.

- Wientroub S *et al.* The clinical use of autologous marrow to improve osteogenic potential of bone grafts in pediatric orthopedics. *J Pediatr Orthop.* 1989; **9:** 186–90.
- Yandow SM *et al.* Autogenic bone marrow injections as a treatment for simple bone cyst. *J Pediatr Orthop.* 1998; **18:** 616–20.

 (d).

Aneurysmal bone cysts can behave like low-grade malignant lesions. Approximately 30% of ABCs are associated with other tumours, most commonly giant-cell tumour. Radiotherapy should not be used, as it may lead to sarcomatous change.

 (e).

Aneurysmal bone cysts most commonly occur in the tibia, they are most commonly eccentric metaphyseal lesions, and they are slightly more common in women. Liquid nitrogen is the most popular form of adjuvant therapy. Radiographs demonstrate a characteristic 'soap-bubble' appearance.

 (a).

This clinical scenario is typical of osteoid osteoma. Osteoid osteoma is a benign skeletal neoplasm of unknown aetiology that is composed of osteoid and woven bone. The tumour is usually smaller than 1.5 cm in diameter. Pain is usually worse at night and is classically relieved by aspirin.

 (b).

Osteoid osteoma is usually associated with few or no systemic symptoms. The tumour produces high levels of prostaglandin E_2, and aspirin is effective for analgesia as it inhibits prostaglandin E_2 synthesis.

 (c).

Enchondroma is a solitary, benign, intramedullary cartilage tumour. It is the commonest primary bone tumour found in the hand.

 (d).

Adamantinoma is a low-grade biphasic tumour of epithelial and osteofibrous origin. It most commonly occurs in the anterior tibial cortex, and is known to metastasise to the lungs.

 (e).

McCune–Albright syndrome in its classic form consists of at least two features of the triad of polyostotic fibrous dysplasia, café-au-lait skin pigmentation and autonomous endocrine hyperfunction. The commonest form of autonomous endocrine hyperfunction in this syndrome is gonadotropin-independent precocious puberty.

 (b).

The condition deteriorates during pregnancy, as the tumour cells have a high number of hormone receptors and become more active in pregnancy.

(A10) (a).

All of the tumours listed are benign, but chondroblastoma and giant-cell tumour are benign tumours which are associated with pulmonary metastasis in rare cases.

(A11) (c).

Osteochondromas account for 20–50% of benign bone tumours and 10–15% of all bone tumours.

(A12) (d).

Osteochondroma lesions do not increase in size after growth plate closure. The male:female ratio is 1.5:1.

(A13) (a).

The risk of malignant transformation is less than 1% for solitary osteochondromas. However, it is 25–30% in multiple osteo-chondromatosis.

(A14) (e).

Hereditary multiple osteochondromatosis is inherited in an auto-somal dominant manner, and most commonly occurs in the first decade of life. The risk of malignant transformation is 25–30%, and sessile lesions carry a higher risk of malignant transformation. A cartilage cap greater than 2 cm in diameter raises the suspicion of malignant transformation.

(A15) (c).

Chondrosarcoma most commonly occurs in the fifth to sixth decade of life, and the male:female ratio is 1.5:1. A better prognosis is seen with clear-cell chondrosarcoma, and only a 10% survival rate is reported for dedifferentiated chondrosarcoma. Patients with Ollier's disease (multiple enchondromatosis) or Maffucci's syn-drome (multiple enchondromas and haemangiomas) are at much higher risk of chondrosarcoma than the normal population, and often present in their third or fourth decade.

(b).

The Ewing's sarcoma family of tumours (ESFT) includes Ewing's sarcoma, peripheral primitive neuroectodermal tumour and neuro-epithelioma, and t (11;22) gene translocations are commonly seen in these tumours.

- Downing JP *et al.* Detection of the (11;22)(q24;q12) translocation of Ewing's sarcoma and peripheral neuroectodermal tumour by reverse transcription polymerase chain reaction. *Am J Pathol.* 1993; **143:** 1294–300.

 (e).

Ewing's sarcoma occurs nine times more commonly in Caucasians. It most commonly occurs in the first and second decades of life. The male:female ratio is 1.5:1. The commonest site of involvement is the femur. Ewing's sarcoma originates from neural crest cells.

 (d).

Secondary fibrosarcoma has not been reported to arise in osteoid osteoma lesions.

 (a).

Approximately 5 cases of osteosarcoma occur per million in adults aged under 20 years.

 (c).

Osteosarcoma most commonly arises in the distal femur. The relative frequency of occurrence is as follows: distal femur, 40%; proximal tibia, 20%; proximal humerus, 10%; pelvis, 8%.

 (b).

Telangiectatic osteosarcoma is a rare and aggressive variant of osteosarcoma. It is often entirely osteolytic on plain radiographs. Bone and cortical destruction are present, as well as periosteal reaction and Codman's triangles.

(A22)   (e).

Patients with elevated alkaline phosphatase values at diagnosis are more likely than others to have pulmonary metastases. Patients without metastases with an elevated lactate dehydrogenase (LDH) level are less likely to do well than those with an LDH level within the reference range.

(A23)   (d).

Transverse incisions require a wider soft tissue resection at the time of definitive surgery, so they are contraindicated. A frozen-section sample should always be sent to verify that a biopsy of the tumour has been taken. Any haematoma around the tumour should be considered contaminated. A large haematoma may dissect the soft and subcutaneous tissues and contaminate the entire extremity, making limb-sparing surgery impossible. The port of entry for the drain has to be in proximity to and in continuity with the skin incision, not to its sides. The drain path is considered to be contaminated, and has to be excised along with the surgical specimen, at the time of definitive surgery.

(A24)   (a).

Tumours that commonly metastasise to bone are those of the thyroid, breast, lung, kidney and prostate. Primary ovarian tumours very rarely metastasise to bone.

- Kumar L *et al.* Bone metastasis in ovarian cancer. *Asia Oceania J Obstet Gynaecol.* 1992; **18**: 309–13.

(A25)   (d).

The Mirels' score is based on the following four parameters: pain, site of lesion, nature of lesion, and amount of cortical involvement of the lesion. A maximum of 3 points can be scored for each parameter, giving a total possible score of 12. A score of 9 is associated with a 33% probability of pathological fracture. Therefore prophylactic fixation has been recommended for lesions that score 8 or more.

- Mirels H. Metastatic disease in long bones. A proposed scoring system for diagnosing impending pathologic fractures. *Clin Orthop Relat Res.* 1989; **249**: 256–64.

Section 11

Extended matching questions

Metabolic bone disease

    (a) Hyperparathyroidism
    (b) Hypoparathyroidism
    (c) Renal osteodystrophy
    (d) Vitamin D resistant rickets
    (e) Familial hypophosphataemic rickets
    (f) Nutritional rickets
    (g) Albright's syndrome
    (h) Fanconi's syndrome
    (i) Hypophosphatasia
    (j) Osteoporosis
    (k) Paget's disease
    (l) Osteopetrosis

For each of the conditions described below, select the most likely diagnosis from the list given above. Each response may be used once, more than once or not at all.

 A condition that results from an abnormality in the parathyroid hormone receptor and is clinically associated with brachydactyly.

(Q2) An autosomal recessive disorder which results in low levels of alkaline phosphatase and is diagnosed by increased levels of urinary phosphoethanolamine.

(Q3) A quantitative defect of bone resulting in decreased bone mass.

(Q4) An X-linked dominant disorder resulting from impaired renal tubular reabsorption of phosphate.

(Q5) A condition resulting from increased osteoclast activity, leading to increased plasma calcium and decreased plasma phosphate levels. It may result in osteitis fibrosa cystica and hyperreflexia.

Answers

(A1) (g).

(A2) (i).

(A3) (j).

(A4) (e).

(A5) (a).

Inflammatory arthritides

(a) Ankylosing spondylitis
(b) Reiter's syndrome
(c) Psoriatic arthritis
(d) Enteropathic arthritis
(e) Adult rheumatoid arthritis
(f) Juvenile rheumatoid arthritis
(g) Systemic lupus erythematosus
(h) Sjögren's syndrome
(i) Scleroderma

For each of the conditions described below, select the most likely diagnosis from the list given above. Each response may be used once, more than once or not at all.

Q6 An oligoarticular condition mainly affecting the small joints of the hands and feet. Clinically swollen digits and nail pitting are present, and 50% of patients are HLA B27 positive.

Q7 A condition characterised by the triad of conjunctivitis, urethritis and oligoarticular arthritis.

Q8 A condition characterised by bilateral sacroiliitis and anterior uveitis with 90% of patients positive for HLA B27. Radiographic features consist of vertebral squaring and vertical syndesmophytes.

Q9 Polyarthritis associated with a malar rash, pancytopaenia, pericarditis and nephritis. Patients are usually positive for antinuclear antibody and HLA DR3.

Answers

A6 (c)

A7 (b).

A8 (a).

A9 (g).

Osteochondroses

(a) Osgood–Schlatter disease
(b) Van Neck's disease
(c) Sinding-Larsen and Johansson syndrome
(d) Sever's disease
(e) Kohler's disease
(f) Panner's disease
(g) Kienbock's disease
(h) Scheurmann's disease
(i) Freiberg's infraction
(j) Thiemann's disease
(k) Blount's disease

For each of the conditions described below, select the most likely diagnosis from the list given above. Each response may be used once, more than once or not at all.

Q10 A 5-year-old boy complains of pain, tenderness and swelling in his left foot. Radiographs demonstrate fragmentation and sclerosis around the navicular.

Q11 A 15-year-old girl complains of pain and swelling in her forefoot. Radiographs demonstrate fragmentation and sclerosis around the second metatarsal head.

(Q12) A 14-year-old boy complains of pain around his right knee. Radiographs demonstrate fragmentation and irregularity around the tibial tuberosity.

(Q13) A 7-year-old boy complains of pain in his left elbow. Radiographs demonstrate fragmentation and irregularity of the capitellum.

(Q14) A 14-year-old boy complains of pain in his knee. He is markedly tender over the inferior pole of the patella, and radiographs confirm fragmentation in this area.

Answers

(A10) (e).

(A11) (i).

(A12) (a).

(A13) (f).

(A14) (c).

Growth plate

   (a)   Secondary bony epiphysis
   (b)   Reserve zone
   (c)   Proliferative zone
   (d)   Maturation zone
   (e)   Degenerative zone
   (f)   Zone of provisional calcification
   (g)   Primary spongiosa
   (h)   Secondary spongiosa

For each of the statements given below, select the zone of the growth plate in which these findings occur, from the list given above. Each response may be used once, more than once or not at all.

(Q15)   Oxygen tension is lowest in this zone and chondrocyte death occurs.

(Q16)   Acute haematogenous osteomyelitis classically affects this zone.

(Q17)   Abnormality of osteoblasts and collagen synthesis in this zone results in osteogenesis imperfecta.

(Q18)   Defects associated with achondroplasia occur in this zone.

Answers

(A15)   (f).

(A16)   (g).

(A17)   (h).

(A18)   (c).

Bone dysplasia

(a)   Achondroplasia
(b)   Spondyloepiphyseal dysplasia
(c)   Multiple epiphyseal dysplasia
(d)   Metaphyseal chondrodysplasia
(e)   Kniest dysplasia
(f)   Achondrogenesis

(g)   Chondrodysplasia punctata
(h)   Progressive diaphyseal dysplasia
(i)   Diastrophic dysplasia
(j)   Hurler's syndrome
(k)   Hunter's syndrome
(l)   Sanfillipo's syndrome
(m)   Morquio's syndrome

For each of the conditions described below, select the most likely diagnosis from the list given above. Each response may be used once, more than once or not at all.

(Q19)   Autosomal dominant, short-trunked, disproportionate dwarfism associated with joint stiffness and contractures. Retinal detachment and myopia are also commonly seen.

(Q20)   Autosomal dominant condition that is the commonest form of disproportionate dwarfism.

(Q21)   Autosomal recessive short-limbed dwarfism associated with a disorder of collagen type II in the physis.

(Q22)   Autosomal recessive form of proportionate dwarfism associated with increased urinary excretion of keratan sulphate.

(Q23)   Sex-linked recessive form of proportionate dwarfism associated with increased urinary excretion of dermatan and heparan sulphate.

Answers

(A19)   (e).

(A20)   (a).

(A21) (i).

(A22) (m).

(A23) (k).

Antibiotic mode of action

(a) Beta-lactams
(b) Aminoglycosides
(c) Macrolides
(d) Tetracyclines
(e) Glycopeptides
(f) Rifampicin
(g) Fluoroquinolones
(h) Sulphonamides

For each of the following mechanisms of action, select the antibiotic group to which it applies from the list given above.

(Q24) Inhibit bacterial peptidoglycan synthesis.

(Q25) Bind to cytoplasmic RNA and inhibit protein synthesis.

(Q26) Inhibit DNA gyrase.

(Q27) Interfere with insertion of glycan subunits into the cell wall.

Answers

(A24) (a).

(A25) (b).

(g).

 (e).

Musculoskeletal infections

(a) *Staphylococcus aureus*
(b) *Staphylococcus epidermidis*
(c) *Streptococcus pyogenes*
(d) Group A Streptococcus
(e) *Pseudomonas aeruginosa*
(f) *Haemophilus influenzae*
(g) *Neisseria gonorrhoeae*
(h) *Borrelia burgdorferi*
(i) *Clostridium tetani*
(j) *Clostridium perfringens*
(k) *Salmonella*

For each of the following clinical scenarios, select which organism is responsible from the list given above.

(Q28) Commonest causative organism for cellulitis.

(Q29) Commonest causative organism in surgical wound infection.

(Q30) Characteristic organism associated with acute monoarticular septic arthritis in sexually active adults.

(Q31) Commonest organism associated with infection of total joint arthroplasty.

(Q32) Characteristic organism associated with osteomyelitis in patients with sickle-cell disease.

Q33 Organism that results in acute self-limiting joint effusions, which is transmitted by tick bites.

Answers

A28 (d).

A29 (a).

A30 (g).

A31 (b).

A32 (k).

A33 (h).

Knee pain

(a) Discoid meniscus
(b) Synovial plica
(c) Osteosarcoma
(d) Parameniscal cyst
(e) Posterior cruciate ligament injury
(f) Anterior cruciate ligament injury
(g) Rheumatoid arthritis
(h) Osteochondritis dissecans
(i) Degenerate meniscal tear
(j) Medial collateral ligament injury
(k) Pigmented villonodular synovitis
(l) Osteoarthritis of the knee

For each of the following clinical scenarios, select the most likely diagnosis from the list given above.

(Q34) A 52-year-old mechanic has a 6-month history of pain and clicking in his right knee. There is no history of trauma. On examination no effusion is present, but medial joint line tenderness is noted.

(Q35) A 25-year-old man complains of intermittent giving way of his left knee. He injured the knee 3 months ago while skiing, and recalls immediate swelling on that occasion. On examination no effusion is present, meniscal provocation tests are negative, but he does have increased translation in the anteroposterior plane.

(Q36) A 15-year-old boy has a 3-month history of pain and swelling in his right knee which comes on after playing football. After resting the pain resolves but the knee continues to feel stiff. On examination a small effusion is present, but no joint line tenderness is noted, and meniscal provocation tests are negative.

(Q37) A 32-year-old woman has an 18-month history of intermittent swelling and stiffness in her left knee. There is no history of trauma prior to the onset of symptoms. On examination there is a large tense effusion in the supra-patellar pouch. Arthrocentesis yields heavily bloodstained synovial fluid.

(Q38) An 8-year-old boy complains of pain in his right knee. The pain is brought on by walking, running or twisting, and is associated with a clunking sensation. On examination, lateral joint line tenderness is noted.

Answers

(A34) (i).

(A35) (f).

(A36) (h).

(A37) (k).

(A38) (a).

Congenital hand disorders

(a) Radial club hand
(b) Ulnar club hand
(c) Cleft hand
(d) Radio-ulnar synostosis
(e) Symphalangism
(f) Camptodactyly
(g) Clinodactyly
(h) Congenital clasped thumb
(i) Syndactyly
(j) Preaxial polydactyly
(k) Postaxial polydactyly
(l) Central polydactyly

For each of the conditions described below, select the most likely diagnosis from the list given above.

(Q39) The commonest congenital hand anomaly.

(Q40) Curvature of the little finger towards the ring finger.

(Q41) Duplication of the thumb.

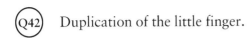

Q42 Duplication of the little finger.

Q43 Absence of the thumb and index finger, associated with shortening of the distal radius.

Answers

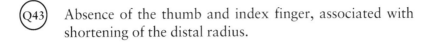

A39 (i).

A40 (g).

A41 (j).

A42 (k).

A43 (a).

Hand lesions

(a) Xanthoma
(b) Neurolemmoma
(c) Neurofibroma
(d) Glomus tumour
(e) Epidermal inclusion cyst
(f) Ganglion
(g) Calcinosis
(h) Osteoid osteoma
(i) Enchondroma
(j) Carpometacarpal boss
(k) Dejerine–Sottas disease
(l) Turret exostosis

For each of the conditions described below, select the most likely diagnosis from the list given above.

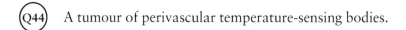

(Q44) A tumour of perivascular temperature-sensing bodies.

(Q45) A painless slow-growing mass arising subsequent to a penetrating injury of the hand.

(Q46) Localised nerve swelling resulting from hypertrophic interstitial neuropathy.

(Q47) Solitary tumour of Schwann cell origin not usually associated with any neurovascular deficit.

Answers

(A44) (d).

(A45) (e).

(A46) (k).

(A47) (b).

Paediatric hip conditions

(a) Developmental dysplasia of the hip
(b) Congenital coxa vara
(c) Legg–Calve–Perthes disease
(d) Slipped upper femoral epiphysis
(e) Proximal femoral focal deficiency
(f) Transient synovitis
(g) Septic arthritis
(h) Avascular necrosis

For each of the conditions described below, select the most likely diagnosis from the list given above.

Q48   A 2-year-old boy is noted to have been limping for the past 2 days. There is no history of trauma, although he is recovering from a recent upper respiratory tract infection. He is apyrexial, and blood tests are within normal limits.

Q49   A 13-year-old girl, who is known to suffer from hypo-thyroidism, has a 2-week history of left knee pain. On examination of the knee no abnormality is noted, but she is found to have obligatory external rotation on hip flexion.

Q50   A 5-year-old boy complains of pain in his hip, and limps when walking. He is noted to have decreased internal rotation and abduction. Radiographs demonstrate frag-mentation of the femoral head.

Answers

A48   (f).
A49   (d).
A50   (c).

Lower limb muscles

(a)   Tibialis anterior
(b)   Tibialis posterior
(c)   Flexor digitorum longus
(d)   Flexor digitorum brevis
(e)   Flexor hallucis longus
(f)   Flexor accessorius
(g)   Adductor hallucis

    (h)   Abductor hallucis
    (i)   Abductor digiti minimi
    (j)   Peroneus longus
    (k)   Peroneus brevis

For each of the muscles described below, select the most appropriate response from the list given above.

(Q51)   The most important muscular supporting structure of the medial longitudinal arch.

(Q52)   The most important supporting structure of the lateral longitudinal arch.

(Q53)   With the foot inverted and in a neutral position, along with the tibialis posterior, this muscle acts as an inverter of the foot.

(Q54)   This muscle initiates heel raising from a standing position.

(Q55)   This muscle assists in maintaining the transverse arch, and is a component of the third layer of the muscles of the sole of the foot.

Answers

(A51)   (e).

(A52)   (j).

(A53)   (a).

(A54)   (b).

(A55)   (g).

Index

Notes: locators in italics indicate 'answers' to questions.